D1760798

OXFORD MEDICAL PUBLICATIONS

# Paediatric Palliative Medicine

# Oxford Specialist Handbooks in Paediatrics

# Paediatric Palliative Medicine

## Richard D.W. Hain

Senior Lecturer in Child Health,
Cardiff University of Medicine,
Consultant and Lead Clinician in Paediatric Palliative
Medicine, Welsh Managed Clinical Network in
PPM Children's Hospital,
Cardiff, UK

## Satbir Singh Jassal

Medical Director,
Rainbows Children's Hospice,
Lark Rise,
Loughborough, Leicestershire, UK

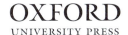

OXFORD
UNIVERSITY PRESS

# OXFORD

UNIVERSITY PRESS

Great Clarendon Street, Oxford OX2 6DP

Oxford University Press is a department of the University of Oxford.
It furthers the University's objective of excellence in research, scholarship,
and education by publishing worldwide in

Oxford  New York

Auckland  Cape Town  Dar es Salaam  Hong Kong  Karachi
Kuala Lumpur  Madrid  Melbourne  Mexico City  Nairobi
New Delhi  Shanghai  Taipei  Toronto

With offices in

Argentina  Austria  Brazil  Chile  Czech Republic  France  Greece
Guatemala  Hungary  Italy  Japan  Poland  Portugal  Singapore
South Korea  Switzerland  Thailand  Turkey  Ukraine  Vietnam

Oxford is a registered trade mark of Oxford University Press
in the UK and in certain other countries

Published in the United States
by Oxford University Press Inc., New York

© Oxford University Press, 2010

British Library Cataloguing in Publication Data
Data available

Library of Congress Cataloging-in-Publication Data
Data available

Typeset by Cepha Imaging Private Ltd., Bangalore, India
Printed in China
on acid-free paper through
Asia Pacific Offset Ltd

ISBN 978-0-19-923632-9

10  9  8  7  6  5  4  3  2  1

# Preface

Palliative medicine in children has emerged as a subspecialty over the last few years. There is an increasing body of expertise and knowledge in the care and management of the child with a life-limiting condition.

The number of specialists in paediatric palliative medicine is increasing. For most children with a life-limiting condition, however, the majority of their care is still provided by professionals without specialist training in palliative medicine. For most of the life of a child with a life-limiting condition, care is provided, not by a palliative care team, but by a general paediatric or other subspecialist team such as oncology, neurology, or cardiology. Others will be cared for by primary care teams, or sometimes by adult palliative medicine teams.

For most of these, having to care for a dying child will nevertheless be a relatively rare event. The aim of this book is to equip them to provide good basic palliative medicine for children in their care despite this lack of training or experience with dying children. Its main use will be among paediatric teams in hospitals, primary care teams (particularly those who are linked to a children's hospice), and community paediatric teams.

Children's palliative medicine encompasses symptom control but is not limited to it. The book also considers the philosophy and models that support delivery of palliative medicine to children and also the communication and coping skills needed by palliative care professionals. The book concludes with a handy formulary containing the drugs most used in paediatric palliative care.

If the authors have succeeded in their aim, the unique significance of this handbook is its practicality and portability and thus its capacity to facilitate practical bedside delivery of effective palliative medicine to children by professionals who have not trained or had experience of caring for the dying child.

Richard D.W. Hain
Satbir Singh Jassal
2010

# Foreword

The UK has led the way in the development of paediatric palliative care with it now attaining its rightful place as a subspecialty of paediatrics. The definitions of what constitutes palliative care, and which patients need it, are not clear. However what is clear is that many children with long term conditions have symptoms which need management. This is not just about care at the end of life. Palliative care should be considered as a thread which runs through the lives of children with long term conditions sometimes being more to the fore than others.

The subject is not one which should be the exclusive preserve of the subspecialist. Children and young people requiring palliative care have a whole variety of diagnoses and are often under the care of other specialists and subspecialists. They are also under the care of their primary care team which in the UK is their General Practitioner and in other parts of the world is a primary care paediatrician. The principles of palliative care for children need to be known by all who care for children and the detail by those who will be intimately involved in their care. Richard Hain is a specialist in the subject, and Satbir Jassal a General Practitoner who also directs a children's hospice. They have brought together their expertise from different ends of the spectrum and provide a comprehensive handbook for all who care for children.

The Handbook should also be of great value to the other members of the multidisciplinary team who care for children and their families.

Palliative care is not just about dying but rather about how to make the best of living during what can be a long and drawn out illness which will end in death sometime.

This new specialist handbook is a major step forward in providing material to help all who care for such children to deal with the issues which arise.

The late Cicely Saunders, pioneer of adult palliative care, said that 'The way patients die lives on in the memories of those left behind'. For children, it is way that they live as well as the way that they die that should live on.

Professor Sir Alan Craft
Emeritus Professor of Child Health
Newcastle University

# Foreword

The distinct discipline of paediatric palliative care has only recently emerged from general paediatrics, modelling itself on adult specialist palliative care.

The death of the child is a particularly tragic circumstance and the disorders leading to death in children had been, until recently, very different to those in adults. Many children are now living with chronic and disabling conditions through childhood and die in their teens or even early adulthood. But that does not mean that paediatric palliative care is emerging too late. On the contrary, the longer period of terminal illness facing children means that the lessons from adult palliative care need to be brought into, and modified in, paediatrics.

Fear of morphine and its related drugs meant that until recently many children were denied adequate analgesia. The evidence for the safe use of adequate analgesia and children has emerged, as has the evidence for use of other drugs and symptom control.

Decision-making is complex, requiring a sound ethical framework and excellent comniunication skills, based around active listening to the child and the parents, never forgetting the other children in the family too.

This book is designed to equip paediatricians and specialist nurses in paediatrics with the knowledge and its evidence base to provide good care at the end of life, whether the child is in their own home or in a hospital or hospice. There are strong arguments for saying that every paediatrician should read such a text whenever they are looking after a dying child; certainly it should be on every departmental bookshelf, at hand to be picked up and opened when it is needed.

It has been said that the way a society cares for its members who are dying reflects the state of civilisation. This is even more true for the way society cares for terminally ill and dying children, teenagers and young people. This book can help improve clinical care at the end of life; in so doing, our society, in one facet, become more civilised.

Professor Baroness Finlay of Llandaff,
FRCP, FRCGP

# Contents

# Detailed contents

# Symbols and abbreviations

| | |
|---|---|
| ► | important |
| ~ | approximately |
| ⌘ | website |
| ACh | acetylcholine |
| ACT | Association for Children with Life-threatening or Terminal Conditions and their Families |
| AIDS | acquired immune deficiency syndrome |
| APLS | advanced paediatric life support |
| BiPAP | bi-level positive airways pressure |
| BNFC | British National Formulary for Children |
| BSPPM | British Society of Paediatric Palliative Medicine |
| CNS | central nervous system |
| CSM | Committee on Safety of Medicine |
| CST | certificate of specialist training |
| $D_2$ | dopamine receptor |
| DEXA | dual-energy X-ray absorptiometry |
| DMD | Duchenne muscular dystrophy |
| DNR | do not resuscitate |
| DSM-IV | Diagnostic and statistical manual |
| EB | epidermolysis bullosa |
| EEG | electroencephalogram |
| FBC | full blood count |
| GABA | γ-aminobutyric acid |
| GAG | glycosaminoglycans |
| GORD | gastro-oesophageal reflux disease |
| GP | general practitioner |
| H1, H2 | two types of histamine receptors |
| HIV | human immunodeficiency virus |
| 5HT | 5-hydroxytryptamine (serotonin; types 5HT1, 5HT2, etc.) |
| IASP | International Association for the Study of Pain |
| ICD | International classification of disease |
| im | intramuscular |
| iv | intravenous |
| MPS | mucopolysaccharide |
| MR | modified release |

| | |
|---|---|
| NCL | neuronal ceroid lipofuscinosis |
| NG | nasogastric |
| NICE | National Institute for Health and Clinical Excellence |
| NIPPV | noninvasive positive-pressure ventilation |
| NMDA | *N*-methyl D-aspartate |
| NSAID | nonsteroidal anti-inflammatory drug |
| OME | oral morphine equivalent |
| OT | occupational therapist |
| $PaCO_2$ | arterial carbon dioxide tension |
| PCA | patient-controlled analgesia |
| PDE | principle of double effect |
| PEG | percutaneous endoscopic gastrostomy |
| PMETB | Postgraduate Medical Education and Training Board |
| po | orally, by mouth *(per os)* |
| PPM | paediatric palliative medicine |
| pr | rectally *(per rectum)* |
| prn | as required *(pro re nata)* |
| RCPCH | Royal College of Paediatrics and Child Health |
| sc | subcutaneous |
| SMA | spinal muscular atrophy |
| SSRI | selective serotonin re-uptake inhibitors |
| SVC | superior vena cava |
| U & E | urea and electrolytes |
| WHO | World Health Organization |

# Philosophy in practice

# Introduction

This chapter will consider:
- a brief history of palliative care in children;
- a definition of palliative care in children;
- how that might need to be worked out in the practical care of children with life-limiting conditions.

# History

The history of the development of children's palliative care is that of a slow evolution over the last 30 years. Since the Second World War medicine has advanced so much and so fast that there seems to be optimism that anything could be healed. This has led many doctors to have difficulties when dealing with children and families where life is limited and treatments are unsuccessful. For many years before the development of the palliative care movement, a lot of good work was done by community and hospital paediatricians, often with very limited resources. The convergence of a number of different threads has acted as a catalyst to the development of paediatric palliative care:

- the recognition of the need for and development of adult palliative care;
- the development of multidisciplinary care at home and in the community by paediatric oncology, and later other paediatric subspecialties;
- the opening of the first children's hospice, Helen House, in 1982 in Oxford UK;
- changing attitudes amongst doctors and nurses towards communication with children and families, in particular recognizing that their wishes on the type and location of care are important;
- an understanding of the importance of team working at health level, but also at social and educational levels.

We have now reached a stage where it has become established that paediatric palliative care is an emerging subspecialty. There are children's hospices being developed in Europe, North America, Australia, and South Africa. In these and other parts of the world, paediatric palliative care is also being provided in hospitals and in the community by paediatricians, family doctors, and adult palliative care doctors. The models of care used are based on the local needs and resources.

Although many children die in the developed world, this is a relatively small number in comparison to the rest of the world. It is vital that we all recognize the need to support the teams working in these underresourced areas of the world. As such we have endeavoured to incorporate advice for these parts of the world in this handbook.

Children are not just small adults. When we manage children we have to understand issues such as:

- differing physiology and pharmacodynamics;
- ethical issues around autonomy and consent;
- changes associated with development and growth;
- family dynamics;
- differing medical conditions, timescales, and symptom presentation;
- intensity of grief and bereavement;
- the limited numbers of life-limited children in developed countries and hence limited experience of the health care professionals.

# Definition

The Royal College of Paediatrics and Child Health (RCPCH) and the Association for Children with life-limiting or terminal conditions and their families (ACT) define palliative care as:

- '… an active and total approach to the care of children, embracing physical, emotional, social and spiritual elements'.[1,2]

So, palliative care is:

- active ( not simply a cessation of treatment);
- total (seeks to address the child's whole experience of symptoms rather than dividing them arbitrarily into physical, emotional, spiritual symptoms).

The American Academy of Pediatrics definition states that paediatric palliative care:

- '… includes the control of pain and other symptoms and addresses the psychological, social or spiritual problems of children and their families'.[3]

While this is similar to the ACT/RCPCH definition, it is perhaps less satisfactory as it suggests that symptom control is a mainly physical phenomenon, somehow separate from psychological, social, and spiritual problems.

# Practical applications

A major dilemma facing paediatric palliative care in the UK currently is identifying which children we should be caring for. This dilemma arises from the following issues.

- Medical intervention often leads to children living longer, e.g. up to 40 years of age with cystic fibrosis and up to 24 years of age with ventilation in Duchenne muscular dystrophy.
- Many children may have severe static neurological problems and not be expected to die in childhood but would still need or benefit from palliative care.
- Predicting life expectancy is notoriously difficult and unreliable in paediatrics.
- A number of neurodegenerative or genetic disorders cannot be identified so, without a label of diagnosis, prognosis becomes unpredictable.

How should the basic principles be put into practice in order to address these issues practically?

From the basic definition, three practical principles can be derived that need to underlie paediatric palliative medicine practice.

- ***Need to balance burden and benefit.*** All interventions in children with life-limiting conditions should plausibly do them more good than harm.
- ***A rational approach is a compassionate one.*** The principles of good medicine are as important in caring for dying children as in paediatrics generally. A rational approach is the way to ensure the best benefit for the least side effects.
- ***Palliative medicine is 'holistic'.*** Palliative care needs to address all the dimensions of a child's experience, not just the physical.

Combining these three principles means that sometimes good palliative medicine will mean balancing physical benefits against (for example) spiritual ones.

# Balance of burden and benefit

For any intervention contemplated:
- there will be a negative impact of some kind or kinds;
- there will also be beneficial effects;
- the first responsibility of the palliative medicine physician is to consider whether the burden to the patient outweighs the benefit;
- it may mean balancing physical benefits against spiritual burdens and vice versa.

*Example* In addressing the possible place of palliative chemotherapy, the potential benefits are:
- the existential value of 'doing something';
- possibility of prolonging the valuable life;
- possibility of relieving pain.

Adverse effects are:
- physical effects of neutropenia;
- need for admission, hair loss, and feeling unwell;
- need for frequent attendances at hospital for drugs and/or blood tests;
- loss of normality.

In considering whether palliative chemotherapy is justified, palliative medicine physicians need to look at physical, psychosocial, and spiritual issues on both sides of the balance.
   This is complicated further.
- The WHO approach provides pain relief for most patients without the need for palliative chemotherapy.
- For some families the process of prolonging life will be, or will be seen as, a process of prolonging death. Not only is prolonging life not a benefit, it may actually be seen as a positive burden.

Decision making in paediatric palliative medicine demands careful and thoughtful consideration of the needs of the individual patient, remembering as far as possible to encompass all dimensions of his or her individual experience. The corollary is that there is no such thing as an intervention that is always inappropriate. It will depend on the individual child's individual experiences at a specific time.

Commencing morphine is sometimes, quite wrongly, considered an automatic response to acknowledgement that treatment is palliative. In reality, the same careful balance needs to be considered.
- Burdens:
  - physical (e.g. constipation);
  - psychosocial (e.g. medicalization);
  - existential/spiritual (e.g. the equation of morphine with impending death).
- Benefits:
  - physical (e.g. relief of physical pain);
  - psychosocial (e.g. relief from dyspnoea);
  - existential/spiritual (e.g. effects of better sleep).

# A rational approach: reforming the 'medical model'

A rational approach is always logical.

An example is the need to make a diagnosis of pain before treating it. The WHO Pain Ladder is the gold standard for managing pain in palliative care. It depends critically on prescribing an appropriate adjuvant at each stage of the ladder. There is a good evidence basis for use of adjuvants, *providing they are used for the appropriate pain syndrome*. It is therefore important to distinguish between pain syndromes on the basis of history and examination findings.

- A rational approach is always evidence-based where possible. Where there is evidence, clearly we must be guided by it if we are to do the best for our patients.
- However, it would not be rational only to do things for which we have a substantial evidence base. The rational response, in the absence of evidence, is to be empirical.

## Evidence-based palliative medicine

The evidence basis in palliative medicine is generally poor, and especially so in the paediatric specialty. Clinical practice in paediatric palliative medicine is underpinned by three levels of evidence.

### Good evidence

See the Cochrane Database. There are relatively few examples, e.g.:
- use of oral morphine;
- WHO Pain Ladder;
- anticonvulsants and antidepressants as adjuvants in neuropathic pain.

### Evidence extrapolated from other contexts

Extrapolation is often from other paediatric specialties such as management of acute pain, or chemotherapy-related nausea and vomiting.

*Example: patient-controlled analgesia (PCA)*
- Little evidence of usefulness in palliative care (adult or paediatric).
- Overwhelming evidence of usefulness in acute pain (adult and paediatric).

Therefore, if the WHO Pain Ladder approach fails, PCA is a logical and rational second-line treatment.

### Little clinical evidence but plausible

Sometimes it is necessary to proceed, not on the basis of evidence, but on the basis that, with a sound understanding of symptom pathophysiology and therapeutics, effectiveness is plausible.

*Example: neuropathic adjuvants in bone pain*
The effectiveness of neuropathic agents in this situation is unproven, but there is a logical sequence.

- Certain adjuvants (including ketamine and gabapentin) are known to be effective in neuropathic pain because of an effect on nerve stimulation.
- It is known that distortion of the microarchitecture of bone results in stimulation of pain receptors.
- It is logical that neuropathic adjuvants may also be effective as an adjuvant in bone pain.
- This is borne out in some laboratory studies.

So, a rational approach would dictate that, while they should not be considered as first-line treatment in bone pain, anti-neuropathic pain agents should be tried if first-line approaches fail.[4] Furthermore, clinical trials should be designed to demonstrate the possibility of a wider use.

## A general approach

More generally, to construct a logical and rational approach (rather than a strictly evidence-based one), we should:

- start with what we know works (e.g. the WHO Guidelines);
- if that fails, use a logical extrapolation from evidence in related areas (e.g. PCA in acute pain);
- if that fails, be creative based on a sound understanding of pharmacology and therapeutics and of laboratory studies (e.g. anti-neuropathic agents in bone pain);
- continually generate well-designed clinical research questions, and trials to answer them.

But:

- We do not have *carte blanche* to use any drug in any way we choose.
- We should always be sceptical of new approaches. It would not serve the interests of our patients if we took at face value the conclusions of 1 or 2 case studies or a visit from a drug rep. Palliative care is particularly vulnerable to the seduction of new approaches because we deal with such a range of symptoms with such a weak evidence base.
- It would be equally wrong to discount new approaches completely. Some will become the standard approach of the future. Fentanyl patches, now the standard second-line approach in palliative care pain, were once novel and untried.

### WHO Pain Ladder

- The WHO Pain Ladder is the gold standard approach to the pain of palliative care in children.
- Although it first appeared in the 1998 publication *Cancer pain relief and palliative care in children*,[5] little in it is specific to cancer pain.
- As pain intensity increases so simple analgesics should give way to simple analgesics with minor opioids such as codeine and, once these no longer control the pain, minor opioids should be discontinued and replaced with major opioids.
- At each stage of the ladder an appropriate adjuvant should be introduced. They should not be delayed until opioids have failed.

# Multidimensionality ('holism')

The third basic principle is that palliative medicine should address all dimensions of a patient's experience. In paediatric palliative care, management of symptoms may be easy. Providing high quality care on the other hand is very difficult. It requires doctors to break out of the traditional pathophysiological paradigm and look at a more holistic problem-solving framework.

Dictionary definitions suggest that holism is: 'the view that a whole system of beliefs must be analysed rather than simply its individual components' and 'the theory of the importance of taking all of somebody's physical, mental, and social conditions into account in the treatment of illness'.

Multidimensionality does *not* mean categorizing a patient's symptoms as 'physical', 'spiritual', or 'psychosocial'. Rather, it means recognizing that all experiences, including symptoms, exist simultaneously in all three dimensions, which must therefore be considered.

- Physical aspects of an experience can be characterized by the questions 'what is happening to me ?' and 'what can be done to stop it?'.
- Psychosocial aspects can be characterized by the questions 'how will this affect my life?' and 'how do I feel about that?'.
- Existential (or spiritual) questions can be characterized by the questions 'why is this happening to me?' and 'what does it mean?'.

In practical terms, a multidimensional or holistic approach means:
- looking at the child, his or her family, and the world around them to determine care;
- looking beyond the physical, at the emotional, spiritual, and environmental;
- accepting that many different professionals may have skills and experience that would benefit the child and to value this diversity of support (Fig. 1.1);
- appreciating the expertise that parents have in looking after their child;
- valuing the support grandparents, family, friends, school, church, and faith can give to the child.

Team working is not easy but is attainable with effort (see Chapters 22 and 23).

## Faced with the reality of a dying child ...

- Don't panic, do not dive in blindly; keep your hands tucked behind your back, your mouth shut, and listen to the parents. In terminal care the parents assume a pivotal role in the care of their child. Only once you have obtained a good history from all sources should you start an examination. Remember the laying on of hands is as important as anything you may discover from your examination. Be methodical, logical, and above all professional: the parents have allowed you into their lives because they perceive that you may be able to help them.
- Once you have formulated a plan of action go through it with the parents in language that they understand. Parents may well feel that they want more or even less than has been recommended to them. Explanation, compromise, and the knowledge that decisions can be

amended as the child's condition changes allow the parents to feel
that they have an informed choice in the care of their dying child. This
particular point is also very important in post-bereavement support.

- Document and disseminate information to all your care team. Check
that they are happy about the care plan and that everyone is clear
about their role.

- Be careful that you do not fall into the same trap as Icarus (who flew
too close to the sun). The intensity of emotion surrounding a dying
child is vast. Many nurses and doctors get so personally attached that
they burn out emotionally. This unfortunately will be of little or no
benefit for the next family they have to look after. Remember to retain
a sensitive professional distance.

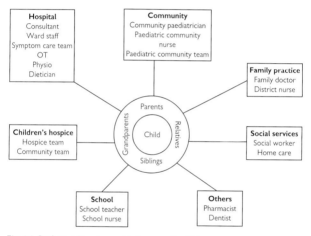

**Fig. 1.1** Professional involvement in the care of a child.

## Summary

Palliative care in children is:
- active—not just a cessation of curative treatment but the active introduction of other approaches
- total—recognizing all dimensions of all experience, particularly symptoms

There are three underlying principles that should always inform management:
- the need to balance and burden and benefit (sometimes need to balance physical benefits against psychosocial or spiritual burdens)
- the need for a rational approach (always logical, evidence-based where possible but empirical where necessary)
- the need for a multidimensional approach, remembering that all experiences occupy all dimensions

## References

**1** ACT/RCPCH (1997). *A guide to the development of children's palliative care services*, 1st edn. Bristol and London: ACT/RCPCH, Bristol and London.

**2** ACT/RCPCH (2003). *A guide to the development of children's palliative care services—updated report*, 2nd edn. ACT/RCPCH, Bristol.

**3** Committee on Bioethics and Committee on Hospital Care (2000). Palliative care for children. *Pediatrics* **106** (2), 351–7.

**4** Colvin, L. and Fallon, M. (2008). Challenges in cancer pain management—bone pain. *Eur. J. Cancer* **44** (8), 1083–90.

**5** World Health Organization (1998). Guidelines for analgesic drug therapy. In *Cancer pain relief and palliative care in children*, pp. 24–8. WHO/IASP, Geneva.

# Models of paediatric palliative care

# Introduction

The UK has a variety of resources for children with life-limiting conditions that is perhaps unrivalled in the world. This is both good and bad. It offers the potential for children and their families to have choices about the location of their care. On the other hand, a multiplicity of agencies brings with it the risk of miscommunication and internecine strife.

The ideal model for providing palliative care to children with life-limiting conditions would offer:
- a choice of location;
- a range of care skills encompassing health care and non-health care, professional and volunteer, specialist and generalist;
- an environment in which it is possible to address a child and family's needs in an unhurried and thorough manner;
- access to medical expertise that includes excellent primary care as well as specialist palliative care for children;
- care that is free at the point of need;
- care that is available to all children with life-limiting conditions.

It is probably impossible for any single agency to provide all these alone. The model is in practice one of cooperation between many different agencies. For this to function effectively requires mutual respect for the services each can provide, and above all good and sensitive inter-professional communication.

Historically, children's palliative care has been influenced largely by four models:
- adult palliative medicine;
- specialist paediatric outreach teams (particularly paediatric oncology);
- children's hospice;
- community paediatric teams.

Each of these has lent its strengths to what we now know as paediatric palliative medicine or children's palliative care.

In considering how palliative care (including palliative medicine) should be delivered to children, there are four questions that should be addressed.
- Who needs it?
- What do they need?
- Who can provide it?
- Where are the children?

# Who needs it?

The early definition of palliative medicine sprang from adults and focused largely on cancer. In 1997, the RCPCH together with ACT addressed this misconception[1,2] by defining four categories of life-limiting conditions in childhood.

## Category I

- Includes children whose condition may be curable, but at diagnosis the possibility of death is significant.
- Examples are cancer and congenital heart disease.
- Of all categories, most closely resembles adult palliative medicine.
- Accounts for approximately one-third of children needing active palliative care at any one time.

## Category II

- Includes children whose disease will certainly kill them prematurely, but only after a period of normality during which they may need no palliative care at all.
- Examples include Duchenne muscular dystrophy, cystic fibrosis.
- Accounts for approximately one-sixth of children needing active palliative care at any one time.

## Category III

- Describes children with conditions whose course is relentlessly progressive from the moment diagnosis is made, if not before.
- Includes metabolic conditions such as mucopolysaccharidosis, Batten's disease, juvenile Huntington's disease.
- Accounts for approximately one-sixth of children needing active palliative care at any one time.

## Category IV

- Includes children with conditions that are not themselves progressive, but whose effects are cumulative over time in such a way as almost inevitably to restrict their lifespan.
- Includes cerebral palsy, severe epilepsy.
- Extraordinarily heterogeneous group, perhaps least like adult palliative care.
- Characterized by extreme unpredictability and numerous 'rehearsals' for a terminal phase before death actually occurs.
- Accounts for at least one-third of children with life-limiting conditions.

The range of life-limiting conditions in childhood is therefore much broader than in the adult specialty, and in particular does not focus on malignant conditions.

The RCPCH/ACT categorization has been the basis for clinical service development and research. It is difficult to validate, however, since the categories describe disease trajectories rather than comprising lists of specific conditions.

# What do they need?

Evidence suggests that the main needs for families are:
- respite;
- multidimensional support for the family;
- service coordination;
- physical symptom management.

# 'Semi-specialist' palliative care for children

## Children's hospice

- Identified by most families as an invaluable resource.
- Typically custom-built facilities, providing excellent environment for multidimensional care.
- Typically house 5–15 children.
- High staff to patient ratio.
- Combines many benefits of hospital, but in a much more 'home-like' environment.
- Main emphasis is on specialist respite.
- Medical needs of children in hospice range from primary care to specialist paediatric palliative medicine. Ideally, therefore, medical support should be available from both GPs and paediatricians.
- Many GPs in children's hospices have undertaken postgraduate training in PPM.
- Increasingly, hospices offer specialist PPM through arrangements with the local tertiary paediatric palliative medicine team.
- Typically little or no statutory funding, so operate independently of Trusts (this independence can be valued by families).
- Provide a wide range of services, often including complementary therapies.
- Most provide these only for their own patients.

Children's hospices offer a unique and greatly valued resource to children with life-limiting conditions. In the UK, we probably have more children's hospices than the rest of the world put together. Their services are usually provided at no cost either to patient or to the Trust. It is very important that paediatricians support hospices and work with them if seamless palliative care for children is to be achieved.

## Specialist paediatric outreach teams

- Originated in oncology, but now includes other subspecialties such as respiratory, gastroenterology, and neonatology.
- Often profound expertise in managing symptoms associated with narrow range of conditions.
- Typically, the outreach team is well known to family from diagnosis, facilitating transition to palliative care if necessary.
- Facilitates care of child by parents at home, often avoiding need for respite admission elsewhere.
- Difficult to maintain skills in the face of new developments in symptom control techniques.
- Depends on medical support from specialist palliative medicine, which is not always easily available.

## Community paediatric teams

- Considerable experience with life-limiting conditions, particularly in RCPCH/ACT categories II, III and IV.
- Symptom control skills increasingly being expected of trainees in community paediatrics and neurodisability.
- Can care for child at home or at school.
- Access to multidisciplinary team, including community physiotherapy, occupational therapy, dietetic and psychology services.

## Adult palliative medicine teams

- Usually profound expertise in symptom control.
- Considerable experience.
- Accessible; currently much more numerous than paediatric specialists.
- Relatively large evidence base for symptom control approaches.
- Should not care for children except in collaboration with a paediatrician.
- Often little experience outside cancer.
- Inpatient units often not suitable for younger children.

Even following recognition of palliative medicine as a paediatric subspecialty in 2009, there is an important role for adult palliative medicine physicians in the care of older teenagers and young adults, and also in advising paediatricians in those many areas where there is no specialist paediatric service available.

# Paediatric palliative medicine

## PPM specialists

- Palliative medicine recognized by PMETB (Postgraduate Medical Education and Training Board) as subspecialty within paediatrics in 2009.
- Currently fewer than 10 consultants in PPM in the UK.
- Most based in tertiary paediatric centres in major cities.
- Liaise with all providers of palliative care to children whenever specialist palliative medicine is required (Fig. 2.1).
- See patients at home, hospital, hospice, school, and in outpatients.

## Paediatrician with special interest in palliative medicine

- Currently between 50 and 60 in the UK.
- Usually have workload in related discipline (especially community paediatrics, paediatric oncology, neurodisability or neurology).
- Currently recognition of 'with interest' status is informal, usually based on acquisition of postgraduate qualification in palliative medicine.
- In future, status of paediatricians 'with an interest' will become more formal.
- Some children's hospice GPs have accumulated similar training and experience. The status of GPs with 'a special interest' will probably also be formalized in the future.

## GPs working in children's hospices

- Medical cover for most children's hospices is through a local GP practice.
- Expert primary care is needed by most children in hospices. Specialist paediatric input is needed by only a proportion.
- There is great variation in experience and training of GP children's hospice doctors. Many have undertaken postgraduate training and can offer considerable support.

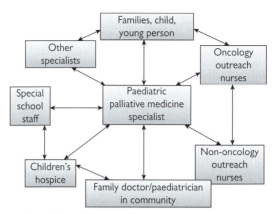

**Fig. 2.1** Role of PPM specialist is to work with and support all agencies providing palliative care for children.

# Where are the children?

- The child with a life-limiting condition spends most of their time at home or at school.
- An ideal model should allow for palliative care to be provided in these environments.
- Admissions to most children's hospices are primarily for respite.
- Death in hospital is common, but it is hard to provide optimal palliative care in an acute paediatric hospital environment.
- Home is the location preferred by most families for death to occur. However, the choice of place of death is very important[3] and many families will choose hospice or hospital instead.
- It appears that around half of children who could benefit from a hospice are never referred.[4]
- It is not clear whether this is because they decide against it, or because it is not offered, or (perhaps more probably) a combination of the two.

## Summary

An ideal model of palliative care would allow:
- expert care to follow the child, wherever the child is
- good access to specialist medical and nursing expertise in palliative care
- choice for family and child of inpatient- or outpatient-based management

This requires a model that is either:
- community-based, reaching into the hospital
- hospital- or hospice-based, reaching out to the home and school; or
- a combination of the two

Given the variety of models that have developed, the last of these is the most common prevailing approach in the UK.

## References

**1** ACT/RCPCH (1997). *A guide to the development of children's palliative care services*, 1st edn. Bristol and London: ACT/RCPCH, Bristol and London.

**2** ACT/RCPCH (2003). *A guide to the development of children's palliative care services—updated report*, 2nd edn. ACT/RCPCH, Bristol.

**3** Vickers, J., Thompson, A., Collins, G.S., Childs, M., and Hain, R. (2007). Place and provision of palliative care for children with progressive cancer: a study by the Paediatric Oncology Nurses' Forum/United Kingdom Children's Cancer Study Group Palliative Care Working Group. *J. Clin. Oncol.* **25** (28), 4472–6.

**4** Hain, R.D. (2005). Palliative care in children in Wales: a study of provision and need. *Palliat. Med.* **19** (2), 137–42.

# Ethics in palliative care

# Introduction

Ethics does not provide a rigid machine for resolution of complex decisions, so that a difficult clinical question can be fed into one end and a correct answer extracted from the other. Neither should the palliative phase be seen as a time when ordinary ethical principles no longer apply and when anything is permissible providing the intention is good.

Ethical principles in palliative medicine are no different from in other medical disciplines. Clinical decisions at the end of life, however, may involve ethical considerations and judgements that are particularly complex and on whose outcome much may depend.

# Review of basic ethical principles

There are four basic medical ethical principles:
- beneficence (an obligation for doctors to do good for their patients);
- non-maleficence (an obligation for doctors to avoid doing harm to their patients);
- autonomy (an obligation for doctors to ensure a patient feels valued and respected as an individual);
- justice (an obligation for doctors to give equal value to their patients).

To these can usefully be added a fifth:[1]
- attention to scope (the obligation to consider the application of these principles to an individual, patient-specific situation).

The underlying principles of palliative medicine (Chapter 1) are:
- the need to balance burden and benefit;
- the need for a rational approach;
- the need for multidimensionality (holism).

It follows that:
- since all palliative interventions carry the possibility of both good and bad effects, the principles of beneficence and non-maleficence require that a judgement be made about the relative risk;
- interventions should be carried out if the potential benefit probably outweighs the potential burden;
- the extent and limitations of evidence in respect of these must be known; the existing evidence base should be accessed by clinicians and utilized in a rational manner;
- both benefits and burdens need to be considered in all dimensions (physical, spiritual, and psychosocial);
- in the absence of possibility of cure, benefits in one dimension may need to be balanced against burdens in another. For some patients on some occasions, this may mean prioritizing quality of life over its duration, or even over the chance for cure;
- since such judgements involve subjective experience, it is necessary to canvass and give weight to the views of child and family in making them;
- service delivery systems may need to be modified to allow equal access by all those who could benefit;
- decision making should be honest, transparent, justifiable, and well-recorded.

# Principle of double effect (PDE)

Double effect is an important principle in palliative care.[2]

- The principle of double effect is that an act is permissible, even if the outcome is undesirable and known beforehand to be possible, providing:
  - the intended act is good;
  - the bad outcome was not the main intention;
  - the good effect is a direct consequence of the action, rather than an incidental consequence of the bad effect;
  - the good effect must be sufficiently desirable to outweigh the bad one.
- PDE recognizes that all interventions have both good and bad effects, and that it is not possible to know with certainty beforehand which will occur.
- It was famously articulated by Catholic moral theologian, Thomas Aquinas, in the thirteenth century, but is a matter of observation and derivable from first principles—there is no casuistry involved.

It therefore follows that:
- The principle of double effect does not equate with, or of itself permit, euthanasia.
- Most prescribing of medications in any context illustrates double effect since there is always the small possibility of an unintended and adverse reaction occurring, for which the prescriber is not morally culpable.
- The principle of double effect is particularly important at the end of life both because prolongation of life may not be a priority, and improvement in life quality assumes a greater importance.

Public perception is sometimes, quite wrongly, that PDE means doctors can and do hasten death through palliative medications. Whilst it has traditionally been uncommon for those working in palliative care to have to justify their clinical decisions and actions in court, this is beginning to change. Fear of litigation should not lead clinicians to become over-cautious, but it is important to ensure that:
- documentation is always clear, dated, and signed;
- all drug doses given are recorded, irrespective of who administers them;
- hospital and primary care records are kept up to date, irrespective of where the child is cared for;
- there is early involvement (if necessary through telephone support) of appropriate professional skills that will usually include specialist paediatrics and palliative medicine as well as primary care;
- any departure from established palliative medicine practice (i.e. the WHO approach, Chapter 4) is documented and justified, especially with respect to opioid initiation, titration, and maintenance.

# Withholding and withdrawing treatment

If:
- 'doing good' means more than simply finding a cure

and
- 'doing harm' is an inevitable part of some treatments,

then it follows that sometimes, balancing burden and benefit, it is in a child's interest to withhold or withdraw medical treatments.[3,4]
  Five situations in which this might be appropriate[4] are as follows.
- The brain dead child. Where criteria of brainstem death are agreed by two practitioners, despite the technical possibility of cardiorespiratory resuscitation.
- Permanent vegetative state. By definition, such a child is unable to react to or relate with the outside world.
- 'No chance' situation. The severity of the child's condition is such that 'life-sustaining' treatment is in reality simply prolonging the process of dying without alleviating suffering.
- 'No purpose' situation. Despite the possibility of long-term survival, it is felt on the child's behalf that the burden of physical or mental impairment is such that it is unreasonable to expect them to bear it. By definition, such a child will never be capable of participating in treatment-related decisions.
- 'Unbearable' situation. The condition is both progressive and irreversible. The child and/or family feel that the burden of further treatment is so great that any potential benefit is irrelevant.

There is evidence[5,6] that, despite these guidelines, inappropriate invasive interventions are still inflicted on children who cannot benefit from them. If it is felt that one of these situations applies:
- ultimately, the key consideration is what is in the child's best interests
- where there is a Trust Clinical Ethics Committee, their opinion should be sought at the earliest opportunity
- any decision to withhold or withdraw curative therapy should be accompanied by consideration of the child's palliative or terminal care needs
- decisions should never be rushed and should be made by the whole team, with all available evidence
- in emergencies, it is often doctors in training who are called on to resuscitate. Life-sustaining treatment should usually be administered and continued until a senior and more experienced doctor arrives. Rigid rules, even for conditions that seem hopeless, should be avoided.
- where there is dissent or uncertainty about whether a clinical situation fits within one of the five categories above, the child's life should be safeguarded by all in health care team in the best way possible.

The legal status of advice given by Trust Clinical Ethics Committees and other professional bodies such as Royal Colleges is largely established by case law and is therefore subject to change. Nevertheless, demonstration of good professional practice will always lend weight to clinical decisions, however ethically challenging. Such good practice includes:

- consistent and clear documentation;
- evidence that the child's and/or family's views have been canvassed and given weight;
- evidence of discussion with colleagues on the health care team;
- reference to published guidelines;
- evidence of discussion with the Clinical Ethical Committee;
- evidence of careful consideration of burden and benefit in all dimensions;
- above all, consistent evidence that the child's own best interests have been made paramount.

## References

**1** Gillon, R. (1994). Medical ethics: four principles plus attention to scope. *Br. Med. J.* **309**, 184–8.

**2** Fohr, S.A. (1998). The double effect of pain medication: separating myth from reality. *J. Palliat. Med.* **1** (4), 315–28.

**3** British Medical Association (1999). *Withholding and withdrawing life-prolonging medical treatment.* [ www.bma.org.uk/news/withdraw.htm]. BMJ Publishing Group.

**4** RCPCH (2004). *Withholding or withdrawing life sustaining treatment in children: a framework for practice,* 2nd edn. RCPCH, Bristol.

**5** Khalil, D., Fardy, C., and Hain, R. (2007). Withholding intensive care in the child who will inevitably die. Primum non nocere—Primum adiuvare! *Welsh Paediatr. J.* **27** (2007), 13–18.

**6** Ramnarayan, P., Craig, F., Petros, A., and Pierce, C. (2007). Characteristics of deaths occurring in hospitalised children: changing trends. *J. Med. Ethics* **33** (5), 255–60.

# Pain: introduction

# Introduction

## Definition

- Pain is: 'an unpleasant sensory and emotional experience associated with actual or potential tissue damage, or described in terms of such damage'.[1]
- A more succinct definition that similarly emphasizes pain's subjective nature is 'pain is whatever the patient says it is'.[2]

The key points in any definition of pain are as follows.
- It is subjective and cannot be properly diagnosed or evaluated using any objective means.
- It is usually interpreted as being the result of tissue damage.
- It is not, in reality, necessarily associated with tissue damage.
- It occurs independently of the child's capacity to express it.

## Classification

There are many systems for classifying pain. They may be based on:
- duration of pain (acute versus chronic);
- intensity (severe, moderate, mild);
- presumed pathophysiology (visceral, somatic, sympathetic mediated)
- location (headache, stomach ache, back ache, etc.)
- sensitivity to opioids.

In palliative medicine, the most widely used classification is pragmatic, based on recognizable clusters of pain symptoms that are associated with response to specific therapeutic interventions:
- neuropathic: characterized by disordered sensation, responsive to adjuvants such as anticonvulsants and antidepressants;
- bone pain: characterized by intense and focal nature, responsive to adjuvants such as nonsteroidal anti-inflammatory drugs (NSAIDs) and bisphosphonates;
- muscle spasm: characterized by responsiveness to muscle relaxants and antispasmodics;
- cerebral irritation: characterized by association with acute brain injury and signs of anxiety, responsive to adjuvants such as benzodiazepines.

Pain is also sometimes considered according to how sensitive it is to opioids:
- opioid sensitive;
- opioid insensitive (or resistant);
- opioid partially resistant.

## Total pain

Total pain describes the concept that pain, of any physical origin or none, occurs in the broader context of an individual's life at that moment.
   This means it is influenced by:
- the severity of any physical tissue damage;
- its impact on function and how the child and/or family feel about it (psychosocial and emotional);
- what pain means to them and any explanations they construct for it (spiritual, or existential).

Attention to one dimension at the expense of the others may be ineffective in alleviating pain.

# Diagnosis, assessment, and evaluation

## Diagnosis

This refers to observing that pain is occurring. Diagnosis of pain in children is complicated by the following facts.

- Younger children may lack the necessary abstract conceptual ability to express it.
- Young children may lack the verbal capacity to express pain.
- Many children, particularly in ACT/RCPCH categories III and IV, are developmentally delayed and may be unable to verbalize.
- Children's experience is often reported by parents or other carers, who may be affected by cultural assumptions such as:
  - children do not suffer pain as intensely as adults;
  - children can and should tolerate pain well;
  - children are vulnerable to the adverse effects of pain killers, such that it is better for them to be in pain than risk toxicity.
- The objective signs of pain are the same as those of other causes of distress, such as anxiety, leading observers to conclude that pain is not the cause.

Where there is doubt it is generally better to assume a child is in pain and treat appropriately, rather than risk allowing them to experience unnecessary discomfort. This can be achieved by:

- recognizing that a child's experience of pain is at least as intense as that of an adult;
- as a default, accepting the word of a parent, nurse, or other carer who knows the child well when they suggest the child may be in pain;
- carefully observing a child's behaviour, or using behaviour-based observational skills routinely (see Chapter 5);
- asking the question 'would I be in pain if this were occurring to me?'

It is rare for families or carers deliberately to overstate a child's pain. If there is doubt, an effective approach is:

- to ask the family member or other carer what behaviour they have observed in the child that leads them to think that they are in pain;
- to record a description of that behaviour carefully;
- to prescribe an appropriate starting dose of an effective analgesic such as an opioid;
- to ask the parent or carer to record over the following week or two whether there has been a reduction in the pain-associated behaviour;
- to review the child a week or two later.

▶ The differential diagnosis here is between pain and other causes of distress, particularly anxiety. Most pain killers are pure analgesics and will have little impact on other causes of distress.

## Assessment refers to a description of the location, quality, timing, and severity of pain. It can be subject to the same complications in children as diagnosing pain (see Chapter 5).

## Evaluation This refers to the measurement of pain severity (see Chapter 5).

# Pharmacological treatment of pain

Management of pain in palliative care differs from pain management in other contexts in the following ways.

- It is usual for there to be more than one source of pain.
- Acute and chronic pain usually coexist.
- Physical pain is complicated by the psychosocial and spiritual context of approaching the end of life.
- Pain is usually gradually increasing in severity. Analgesia in palliative medicine is usually characterized by the need to titrate ever upwards at a carefully considered rate.
- The balance between the benefit of a medication or other intervention against its burden needs to be considered in terms of the immediate quality of life, rather than any long term considerations.

Palliative pain management in children differs from that in adults for the following reasons.

- Children are often relatively resilient to dose-limiting side effects (e.g. confusion).
- Children needing palliative medicine are rarely ward inpatients. Enabling them to remain in a home or home-like environment has a high priority.
- A high priority must be given to avoiding needles when considering which formulations to choose.
- The range of opioids for which safety information is available in children is relatively limited.
- Palliative medicine in children is usually in collaboration with other paediatricians, and preference often needs to be given to medications that are familiar to paediatricians.

As a result of this, the approach to pain management in children is different in a number of ways.

- Neurolytic procedures are rarely justified.
- Buccal and transdermal preparations are preferred where available.
- Opioids for which evidence of safety and effectiveness is limited should be avoided (such as oxycodone). (Table 4.1 indicates some common errors in prescribing major opioids to children.)

Nevertheless, underlying principles remain the same. Safe and effective management of pain in children is ensured by understanding of:

- the individual pain;
- the individual child;
- the pathophysiology of pain;
- a graduated approach to pain management (see Chapter 4, WHO pain guidelines, p. 40).

**Table 4.1** Common errors in prescribing major opioids to children

| Errors | Consequences |
| --- | --- |
| Prescribing major opioids 'as needed' (prn) without background regular major opioids | No background tolerance to adverse effects, particularly drowsiness |
| | Reduced effectiveness and increased toxicity of prn doses, due to metabolic considerations |
| | Rapid fluctuations in serum opioid levels, so therapeutic levels reached only occasionally |
| Wrong dosage interval for oral morphine (e.g. 6 hourly rather than 4 hourly) | Serum concentrations of opioid fall below therapeutic level resulting in breakthrough pain |
| Inappropriate dose of breakthrough opioid relative to regular opioid | The dose of breakthrough opioid should usually be one-sixth of the total daily dose of background regular opioid (see Chapter 7) |
| | If the breakthrough dose is too high, tolerance to adverse effects has not developed and toxicity, particularly drowsiness, will result |
| | If the dose is too low, it will simply be ineffective because of tolerance to analgesia caused by the background opioid dose |
| Over-rapid titration of opioids | If the dose of opioids is increased too quickly, there is no time for tolerance to adverse effects to develop. Providing the patient has free access to breakthrough doses of opioid, 48 hourly review is usually sufficient and allows titration to be done safely and effectively |
| Too early conversion to long-acting opioid | Converting to a long-acting opioid should usually be deferred until the opioid requirements have been stable for some days |
| | Titration of MST® or fentanyl patches, for example, is constrained to some extent by the formulations available |
| Inaccurate opioid rotation | Opioid rotation is a specialist palliative medicine skill |
| | Although it is usually possible to exchange one major opioid for another, the exact equivalent dose will depend on a variety of factors including which drugs they are, how many breakthroughs have been required by the patient, co-prescribed medications, and co-morbidities, particularly renal function |
| | Furthermore, the phenomenon of incomplete cross-tolerance means that unexpected toxicity can occur even when substituted with exactly equipotent doses |

Modified from WHO Guidelines for analgesic drug therapy. Cancer Pain Relief and Palliative Care in Children. Geneva: WHO/IASP;1998.

# WHO pain guidelines

The WHO analgesic ladder[3] (Fig 4.1) is an illustration that, as pain intensity increases, there should be a parallel and appropriate increase in the potency of analgesics used.

## Step 1 (for mild pain)

Simple analgesia, such as:
- paracetamol (acetaminophen);
- aspirin.

## Step 2 (for moderate pain)

Minor opioids such as:
- codeine;
- tramadol (▶ has additional non-opioid analgesic effects);
- low dose buprenorphine patch.

Drugs at step 2 should be added to those already used in step 1.

## Step 3 (for severe pain)

Major opioids such as:
- morphine (first line)
- diamorphine;
- fentanyl;
- high dose buprenorphine patch;
- methadone;
- hydromorphone.

Evidence for other opioids in PPM is either lacking (e.g. oxycodone) or indicates that the risk outweighs the benefit (e.g. pethidine).
    Medications at step 3 should replace those on step 2.

### Adjuvants

At all steps, an adjuvant should be introduced as soon as the nature of the pain is clear. Adjuvants could include the following.
- For neuropathic pain, anticonvulsants (e.g. gabapentin, carbamazepine), antidepressants (particularly amitriptyline), and NMDA receptor antagonists (such as methadone and ketamine).
- For bone pain, NSAIDs, bisphosphonates (e.g. pamidronate), and radiotherapy.
- For muscle spasm, muscle relaxants such as benzodiazepine, baclofen, tizanidine, and botulinum toxin.
- For cerebral irritation, anxiolytics such as benzodiazepines or phenobarbital.
- Steroids can be useful in managing inflammatory mediated pain or pain mediated by oedema round a tumour.
- Chemotherapy. Some chemotherapeutic agents, particularly oral etoposide and vincristine, can reduce the size of a tumour enough to relieve symptoms, without themselves causing major side effects.

### 'Golden rules'

- Always use oral formulations where possible.
- Use appropriate adjuvants at all stages.

- Do not rotate medications within a step, but move on to the next step if pain is no longer controlled (the exception, of course, is at Step 3).
- Major opioids should never be prescribed solely 'as needed'. They should always accompany background major opioids given regularly. See Table 4.1.

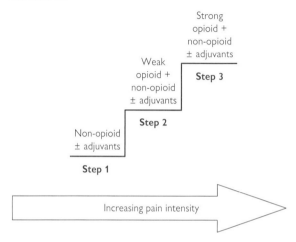

**Fig. 4.1** WHO pain ladder (adapted from reference 3). Modified from World Health Organization Guidelines for analgesic drug therapy, Cancer Pain Relief and Palliative Care in Children. Geneva: WHO/IASP; 1998, pp. 24–8.

## Summary

- Pain is a subjective and multidimensional phenomenon
- Diagnosis, assessment, and evaluation of pain are all complicated in children by the range of diagnoses, developmental levels, and by cultural influences
- Management of pain in palliative care overlaps with, but is different from, management of acute or chronic pain
- Management of pain in children overlaps with, but is distinct from, management of pain in adults
- The basic principles of management of pain in palliative care of adults with cancer can be extrapolated reasonably to the care of children with life-limiting conditions
- The WHO pain ladder is the basis of managing pain in palliative care for children
- The nature of the paediatric specialty means that the implementation of this approach needs to be modified to make it appropriate for children.

### References

**1** IASP Task Force on Taxonomy (1994). Part III: Pain terms, a current list with definitions and notes on usage. In *Classification of chronic pain*, 2nd edn (ed. H. Merskey and N. Bogduk), pp. 209–14. IASP Press, Seattle.

**2** McCaffery, M. and Moss, F. (1968). [Nursing intervention for bodily pain.] *Sogo Kango* **3** (2), 49–58.

**3** World Health Organization (1998). Guidelines for analgesic drug therapy. In *Cancer pain relief and palliative care in children*, pp. 24–8. WHO/IASP, Geneva.

# Pain evaluation

# Introduction

Pain is a subjective phenomenon. It is different for each individual who experiences it, and for any individual will depend on a multiplicity of factors including its cause, context, and meaning. The degree of tissue damage is only one factor among many that contribute to perception of a painful experience. Pain is modulated by complex neurological, biochemical, and psychological influences at many different levels from the periphery to the cortex. Even the 'wiring' of the system itself is subject to change, particularly during childhood. This may result from previous pain experience. The sensation of pain is therefore influenced by innumerable factors, not only at the time of the stimulus, but during the individual's prior experience.

A distinction is sometimes made between 'assessment' and 'measurement' of pain. Measurement refers specifically to quantification of pain, i.e. how severe it is. Assessment describes the broader diagnosis and estimation of a pain experience. Scales that simply quantify pain may not also adequately describe it.

Appropriate tools can report aspects of pain experience. Across childhood, changing developmental levels mean it may be necessary to select from a range of tools in order to assess and measure pain effectively. All children receiving analgesics should ideally be subject to routine assessment of their pain. That this is not usually done is partly a result of the traditionally low priority given to pain in children, but the problem is compounded by scales that are:
- difficult to use;
- uninteresting to children;
- unwieldy for staff.

Selecting the right scale is important, but a scale that is highly validated and eminently suitable for research may be simply too cumbersome for day to day clinical use.

# Characteristics of a pain scale

The ideal pain scale should have the following characteristics.

- Practical. It must capture a child's imagination and be fun to use, as well as simple and quick for staff to administer.
- Appropriately validated. A scale should measure the right phenomenon. Scales measuring physiological responses to pain do not distinguish between pain and anxiety. Since the purpose of a pain scale is to decide on analgesic therapy, a pain scale should measure the symptom that can be treated using analgesics.
- Appropriately applied. Some pain scales have been developed for specific clinical situations. It should not be assumed they will be equally valid in others. For example, scales measuring acute pain are unlikely to be equally valid in measuring chronic pain. This is particularly true of scales relying on behavioural observations, which are often based on patterns derived during specific procedures.
- Developmentally appropriate. No single pain scale is valid across all age groups. Since pain is subjective, and subjective experience needs to be reported by an individual, it is essential that a scale should allow the child to self report where possible.
- Culturally appropriate. Because pain is reported as a subjective phenomenon, the use of language is potentially very important. The use of culturally specific terms (e.g. 'ouchie' in the US) limits usefulness. Scales relying on facial expression should either be racially neutral or be available for different racial groups.

## Special groups

### Neonates and infants[1,2]

Generally unsatisfactory but important measures:

- physiological measures of autonomic function;
- biochemical measures (cortisol, endorphins);
- behavioural measures (nature of cry, facial expression, flailing of arms and legs).

### Children with developmental delay

- Important as pain is a consistent feature.
- Many children are capable of a degree of expression of subjective pain.
- Parents or carers become expert in recognizing pain behaviours and should be believed when they report it.
- Some pain behaviours are common to many children and have been described and correlated with objective measures.[3,4]
- Therapeutic trial of analgesic may be necessary to demonstrate presence or absence of pain.

## Classification of pain scales

There are, in fact, many different pain scales available for children.[5-8] They match this ideal to a greater or lesser extent. They fall into five categories:

- visual analogue self-report scales;
- descriptive self-report scales;
- objective measures of pain;
- behavioural measures;
- multidimensional pain scales.

# Self-report scales

## Visual analogue self-report scales

The most direct means of assessing pain in a child may simply be to ask 'how much does it hurt?' Providing there is an appropriate tool to quantify it, most children have the necessary abstract ability to respond to this. There are many such tools.

### Under six years old

*Faces scale[5,9–11]*

A self-report scale comprising a range of expressions from smiling broadly to crying inconsolably.
- Strengths:
  - attractive;
  - simple;
  - quick to administer.
- Weaknesses
  - faces might equally express mood rather than pain;
  - expressions depict response to acute rather than chronic pain.

*The Oucher[10,12–24]*

Refinement of the Faces scale, using photographs of real faces linked to numerical visual analogue scale 0–100.
- Strengths:
  - well designed;
  - rigorously validated;
  - can be used over a wide range of ages due to a combination of photos and numerical index;
  - race-appropriate alternatives are available.
- Weakness: expressions are those of acute pain rather than chronic.

*Poker chip tool[25–27]*

This uses red plastic poker chips representing 'pieces of hurt', allowing children to choose from 1 ('a little bit of hurt') to 4 ('a lot of hurt').
- Strengths
  - very attractive to children;
  - simple;
  - widely culturally applicable;
  - has been validated.
- Weakness: limited range of responses available.

*Colour scales[28–30]*

An outline of a child's body that a child can colour in using pens or crayons. The child first selects which colours will represent 'worst hurt' and which represent 'no hurt at all'.
- Strengths
  - quickly engages a child's interest;
  - fun to complete;
  - allows expression of feelings of pain;
  - allows child to describe exact site of pain.
- Weakness relatively poorly validated.

*Other scales* There are many other variations on the theme of a visual analogue scale,[30] including:
- a glasses scale;
- ladder scale;
- line scale.

### Six years to adolescence

Many of the analogue scales designed for younger children can be used in this age group as well. Scales developed in adults become increasingly appropriate as the child approaches adolescence. Most are based on a visual analogue scale.

- Strengths
  - well validated in adults;
  - often validated in children;
  - simple to use;
  - quick to administer.
- Weaknesses
  - can only measure one dimension of pain at a time (usually intensity).
    ▶ A broader assessment can be made using a visual analogue scale to quantify an additional dimension such as 'the degree of unpleasantness of pain';
  - may be less valid for chronic pain due to functional habituation (a child may simply forget what it was like not to be in pain).

## Descriptive self-report scales

Since pain is a subjective phenomenon, the child's own description of the nature and severity of their pain is ultimately what needs to be assessed.[31] There are many descriptive self-report scales.[5–8]

- Strengths:
  - accesses subjective experience of pain;
  - based on well validated concept in adults;
  - further validated in children.
- Weaknesses:
  - pain descriptors are known to be influenced by age;
  - labour-intensive, making it difficult to use in clinical situations;
  - original descriptors derived from acute pain, but validated in children with chronic pain.

# Objective and behavioural measures of pain

## Objective measures of pain

The phrase appears inherently contradictory since pain is a subjective experience. Objective assessments can be made, however, of the effect of pain on some measurable physiological parameter.

*Strengths*
- Easy for staff to carry out routinely.
- Independent of developmental stage or capacity to communicate.

*Weaknesses*
- Take no account of emotional, psychological, or spiritual aspects of pain.
- Do not distinguish between pain and other causes of distress.
- Do not allow subjective report of pain experience.

These weaknesses mean that purely physiological parameters are no longer acceptable assessments for children's pain. However, they remain important where there is no alternative, e.g. in some neonatal contexts.

Physiological parameters may, however, add to the discriminatory power of other scales.[32]

## Behavioural measures of pain[3–6,18,21,33–36]

In children under 3 years, communication is not primarily verbal, but uses nonverbal behaviour patterns. Behavioural scales formalize observation of behaviour patterns associated with pain. They allow interpretation of a child's communication of subjective experience. They are not therefore objective measures, although they rely on observation. Since 'body language' remains a feature of communication at all ages, all groups of children and adults (particularly those with impaired cognitive function such as cerebral palsy or neurodegenerative conditions) may also use these.

*Strengths*
- Allow interpretation of subjective pain experience by observer.
- Do not depend on child's willingness to participate.
- Potentially can be used for most developmental stages.
- By identifying appropriate behaviour patterns, can be equally valid for acute and chronic pain.
- By identifying appropriate behaviour patterns, can be used for children with impaired cognition or ability to communicate.

*Weaknesses*
- Often labour-intensive and unwieldy to use in clinical practice.
- Appropriate application is determined by derivation of behaviour patterns. For example, behaviour patterns associated with pain due to procedures may not be seen in chronic cancer pain.
- Some behaviours are age-dependent.

# Multidimensional scales

There are scales that combine aspects of different categories of pain scale. These often include a physiological parameter with some behavioural observation.

Multidimensional pain scales share the strengths and weaknesses of the types of scale on which they draw. They may be of particular value in assessing pain in infants or in chronic pain.

### QUEST approach to managing pain in a child[37]

- Question the child
- Use pain-rating tools
- Evaluate behaviour
- Sensitize parents (i.e. ask them to report the child's pain)
- Take action (i.e. prescribe appropriate analgesic intervention)

# References

**1** Holsti, L. and Grunau, R.E. (2007). Initial validation of the Behavioral Indicators of Infant Pain (BIIP). *Pain* **132** (3), 264–72.

**2** Holsti, L., Grunau, R.E., Whifield, M.F., Oberlander, T.F., and Lindh, V. (2006). Behavioral responses to pain are heightened after clustered care in preterm infants born between 30 and 32 weeks gestational age. *Clin. J. Pain* **22** (9), 757–64.

**3** Hunt, A., Goldman, A., Seers, K., Crichton, N., Mastroyannopoulou, K., Moffat, V., *et al.* (2004). Clinical validation of the paediatric pain profile. *Dev. Med. Child Neurol.* **46** (1), 9–18.

**4** Hunt, A., Wisbeach, A., Seers, K., Goldman, A., Crichton, N., Perry, L., *et al.* (2007). Development of the paediatric pain profile: role of video analysis and saliva cortisol in validating a tool to assess pain in children with severe neurological disability. *J. Pain Symptom Manage.* **33** (3), 276–89.

**5** von Baeyer, C.L. (2006). Children's self-reports of pain intensity: scale selection, limitations and interpretation. *Pain Res. Manag.* **11** (3), 157–62.

**6** von Baeyer, C.L. and Spagrud, L.J. (2007). Systematic review of observational (behavioral) measures of pain for children and adolescents aged 3 to 18 years. *Pain* **127** (1–2), 140–50.

**7** Franck, L.S., Greenberg, C.S., and Stevens, B. (2000). Pain assessment in infants and children. *Pediatr. Clin. North Am.* **47** (3), 487–512.

**8** Hain, R.D. (1997). Pain scales in children: a review. *Palliat. Med.* **11** (5), 341–50.

**9** Hicks, C.L., von Baeyer, C.L., Spafford, P.A., van Korlaar, I., and Goodenough, B. (2001). The Faces Pain Scale–Revised: toward a common metric in pediatric pain measurement. *Pain* **93** (2), 173–83.

**10** Luffy, R. and Grove, S.K. (2003). Examining the validity, reliability, and preference of three pediatric pain measurement tools in African–American children. *Pediatr. Nurs.* **29** (1), 54–9.

**11** McGrath, P.A., Seifert, C.E., Speechley, K.N., Booth, J.C., Stitt, L., and Gibson, M.C. (1996). A new analogue scale for assessing children's pain: an initial validation study. *Pain* **64** (3) 435–43.

**12** Beyer, J.E. (2000). Judging the effectiveness of analgesia for children and adolescents during vaso-occlusive events of sickle cell disease. *J. Pain Symptom Manage.* **19** (1), 63–72.

**13** Beyer, J.E., Denyes, M.J., and Villarruel, A.M. (1992). The creation, validation, and continuing development of the Oucher: a measure of pain intensity in children. *J. Pediatr. Nurs.* **7** (5), 335–46.

**14** Beyer, J.E. and Knott, C.B. (1998). Construct validity estimation for the African–American and Hispanic versions of the Oucher Scale. *J. Pediatr. Nurs.* **13** (1), 20–31.

**15** Beyer, J.E., McGrath, P.J., and Berde, C.B. (1990). Discordance between self-report and behavioral pain measures in children aged 3–7 years after surgery. *J. Pain Symptom Manage.* **5** (6), 350–5.

**16** Beyer, J.E., Turner, S.B., Jones, L., Young, L., Onikul, R., and Bohaty, B. (2005). The alternate forms reliability of the Oucher pain scale. *Pain Manag. Nurs.* **6** (1), 10–17.

**17** Huth, M.M., Broome, M.E., and Good, M. (2004). Imagery reduces children's post-operative pain. *Pain* **110** (1–2), 439–48.

**18** Jacob, E., Miaskowski, C., Savedra, M., Beyer, J.E., Treadwell, M., and Styles, L. (2007). Quantification of analgesic use in children with sickle cell disease. *Clin. J. Pain* **23** (1), 8–14.

**19** Jordan-Marsh, M., Yoder, L., Hall, D., and Watson, R. (1994). Alternate Oucher form testing: gender, ethnicity, and age variations. *Res. Nurs. Health* **17** (2), 111–18.

**20** Knott, C., Beyer, J., Villarruel, A., Denyes, M., Erickson, V., and Willard, G. (1994). Using the Oucher developmental approach to pain assessment in children. *Am. J. Matern. Child Nurs.* **19** (6), 314–20.

**21** Lyon, F. and Dawson, D. (2003). Oucher or CHEOPS for pain assessment in children. *Emerg. Med. J.* **20** (5), 470.

**22** Peden, V. and Saddington, C. (2001). Using the Oucher Scale. Paediatr. Nurs. 13 (3), 24–6.

**23** Sparks, L. (2001). Taking the "ouch" out of injections for children. Using distraction to decrease pain. *Am. J. Matern. Child Nurs.* **26** (2), 72–8.

**24** Yeh, C.H. (2005). Development and validation of the Asian version of the oucher: a pain intensity scale for children. *J. Pain* **6** (8), 526–34.

**25** Cheng, S.F., Hester, N.O., Foster, R.L., and Wang, J.J. (2003). Assessment of the convergent validity of pain intensity in the Pain Sensory Tool. *J. Nurs. Res.* **11** (2), 93–100.

**26** Hester, N.K. (1979). The preoperational child's reaction to immunization. *Nurs. Res.* **28** (4), 250–5.

**27** Suraseranivongse, S., Montapaneewat, T., Manon, J., Chainchop, P., Petcharatana, S., and Kraiprasit, K. (2005). Cross-validation of a self-report scale for postoperative pain in school-aged children. *J. Med. Assoc. Thailand* **88** (3), 412–18.

**28** Eland, J.M. (1981). Minimizing pain associated with prekindergarten intramuscular injections. *Issues Comprehens. Pediatr. Nurs.* **5**, 361–72.

**29** Oztas, N., Ulusu, T., Bodur, H., and Dogan, C. (2005). The wand in pulp therapy: an alternative to inferior alveolar nerve block. *Quintessence Int.* **36** (7–8), 559–64.

**30** Wong, D.L. and Baker, C.M. (1988). Pain in children: comparison of assessment scales. *Pediatr. Nurs.* **14** (1), 9–17.

**31** Varni, J.W., Thompson, K.L., and Hanson, V. (1987). The Varni/Thompson Pediatric Pain Questionnaire. I. Chronic musculoskeletal pain in juvenile rheumatoid arthritis. *Pain* **28** (1), 27–38.

**32** Jay, S.M., Ozolins, M., Elliott, C.H., and Caldwell, S. (1983). Assessment of children's distress during painful medical procedures. *Health Psychol.* **2**, 133–47.

**33** Gauvain-Piquard, A., Rodary, C., and Lemerle, J. (1988). L'atonie psychomotrice: signe majeur de douleur chez l'enfant de moins de 6 ans. *J. Parisiennes Pediatr.* 249–52.

**34** Gauvain-Piquard, A., Rodary, C., and Lemerle, J. (1991). Une echelle d'evaluation de la douleur du jeune enfant: l'echelle DEGR. *J. Parisiennes Pediatr.* 95–100.

**35** Gauvain-Piquard, A., Rodary, C., Rezvani, A., and Lemerle, J. (1987). Pain in children aged 2–6 years: a new observational rating scale elaborated in a pediatric oncology unit—preliminary report. *Pain* **31** (2), 177–88.

**36** Gauvain-Piquard, A., Rodary, C., Rezvani, A., and Serbouti, S. (1999). The development of the DEGR(R): A scale to assess pain in young children with cancer. *Eur. J. Pain* **3** (2), 165–76.

**37** Baker, C.M. and Wong, D.L. (1987). Q.U.E.S.T.: a process of pain assessment in children (continuing education credit). *Orthop. Nurs.* **6** (1), 11–21.

# Pain: steps 1 and 2

# Introduction

There is a tendency for clinicians to be overcautious in their prescription of strong analgesics, probably for the following reasons.
- Most clinicians are not familiar with most of the available analgesics.
- There are a number of medical cultural myths, including:
  - children feel pain less intensely than adults;
  - children are generally vulnerable to the adverse effects of analgesics;
  - it is unnecessary to use an evidence-based approach in the palliative phase;
  - distraction (e.g. using sucrose solution), anxiolysis (e.g. benzodiazepines), or inducing sleep (e.g. chloral hydrate) are acceptable alternatives to analgesia.
- The 'precautionary principle' that the small risk of a serious adverse effect should outweigh the certainty of untreated pain.

The result is a tendency for children to receive inadequate analgesia, either by being prescribed medications that are too weak, or doses that are too low.

The basic principle underlying appropriate management of pain in palliative care is that the benefits of the proposed treatment, measured in terms of quality of life, should always outweigh its burdens. It is therefore essential to know both the desirable and the adverse effects that are anticipated from a medication.

It is usually possible to find an optimal way of prescribing strong analgesics so that the risk of adverse effects remains small while the chance of significant benefit is maximized. This can be achieved by considering:
- which drug to choose;
- the dose of the drug;
- the route of the drug;
- the dosage interval;

These in turn depend on variables within the patient:
- age;
- prior medication, particularly of analgesics such as opioids;
- concurrent illness;
- what has worked previously in that individual patient;
- nature of the pain, including non-physical factors.

It is quite possible for the same dose of the same drug to be prescribed to two patients who are physically very similar with two very different outcomes (see Chapter 3, Principle of double effect (PDE), p. 30).

It is therefore essential that clinicians demonstrate a rational and ideally evidence-based approach to the initiation and escalation of analgesics for pain in palliative care. Departure from this approach risks:
- undertreating pain;
- causing unnecessary adverse effects;
- accusations of professional misconduct such as hastening death.

The WHO guidelines[1] provide the current 'gold standard' in palliative medicine. Departure from the guidelines should be justified and carefully recorded for professional and potentially medicolegal reasons.

They are based on the following principles.
- As pain increases, more potent classes of analgesia should be introduced.
- As a corollary, rotating between drugs of the same potency should not delay introduction of stronger analgesics.
- Certain classes of medications can modulate certain specific types of pain, although they are not primarily analgesics. This defines the term 'adjuvant'.

In the WHO Pain Ladder there are 3 steps (see WHO pain guidelines, p. 40, and Fig. 4.1, p. 41).
- Each step contains analgesics of comparable potency.
- All medications should be given orally wherever possible.
- Adjuvants appropriate for the nature of the pain should be added at each step as necessary.
- Medications on step 2 are added to those in step 1, not substituted.
- Medications on step 3 replace those on step 2. It is rarely appropriate to combine medications on step 2 and step 3.
- There are some inconsistencies, e.g. there is no pharmacological reason for the 'minor opioid' step (step 2).

# Step 1

Analgesics on step 1 are described as 'simple analgesics'. They include aspirin and paracetamol (= acetaminophen in North America).

- Aspirin is rarely used because of concerns about Reye syndrome though it may have a role for children in palliative care in whom this risk is negligible.
- Even at step 1, a diagnosis should be made of the pain (see Chapter 8), and an appropriate adjuvant prescribed.
- Step 1 medications are usually given 'as needed'. If they are needed regularly, it is an indication to move to step 2.

# Step 2

Step 2 medications include 'minor' or 'weak' opioids. In practice, there are three such medications commonly used:
- codeine;
- tramadol;
- buprenorphine at low dose.

## Codeine

- Potency relative to oral morphine (oral morphine equivalent; OME): 0.1.
- Codeine is a precursor of morphine.
- It is effectively a prodrug, converted in the liver to morphine.
- 10–30% of the population cannot convert it. In these patients, codeine is useless. Codeine and tramadol are converted to active forms by the same enzyme. Non-responders to codeine will not benefit from the opioid actions of tramadol, but tramadol's other mechanisms may offer analgesia in some.
- Many patients prefer codeine as it carries less of a stigma than stronger opioids.
- Compared with morphine, codeine is probably more constipating relative to the degree of analgesia.
- Saturation of the liver enzyme and/or intolerable side effects can impose a *de facto* 'ceiling effect'. This is not a true pharmacological ceiling effect as receptor occupancy is not full (see Buprenorphine, p. 61).
- Considerable evidence for safety and effectiveness of codeine in children.
- Not a controlled drug in the UK.

The usefulness of codeine is limited by its pharmacogenetics and its potential to cause constipation. Pharmacologically, a small dose of morphine is preferable to a large dose of codeine. Children and their families, however, often find codeine more acceptable.

## Tramadol

- Tramadol is a derivative of codeine.
- OME 0.2, but effective potency greater than this due to non-opioid analgesic effects via modulation of GABAergic, noradrenergic, and serotonergic systems.
- No evidence of specific benefit in neuropathic pain, though NMDA antagonism has been suggested.
- Very poorly tolerated in a minority of patients due primarily to hypotension.
- Favoured by some patients as it is not a major opioid or a controlled drug in the UK.
- Evidence for safety and effectiveness in acute pain in children.
- No evidence of effectiveness and safety in chronic or palliative care pain.

The role of tramadol in paediatric palliative care has yet to be determined and is probably limited. It can provide a useful 'bridge' between steps 2 and 3, since its non-opioid analgesic properties make it more potent than codeine although it is technically a minor opioid and is not a controlled drug. This can be important to older children, such as boys with Duchenne muscular dystrophy, who are likely to need to be on the medication for a long time and want to avoid as long as possible the stigma of major opioids.

## Buprenorphine

- OME 60.
- Semisynthetic opioid.
- Available sublingually for immediate release.
- Available by transdermal patch for slow release.
- Buprenorphine demonstrates genuine pharmacological 'ceiling effect' but only at higher doses than those usually used clinically.
- Partial agonist; therefore theoretically lower risk of some adverse effects, e.g. respiratory depression, constipation.
- For the same reason, harder to reverse using naloxone if needed.
- Considerable evidence of safety and effectiveness in some forms of pain in children.
- Little systematic evidence of effectiveness and safety in palliative care.

Buprenorphine potentially has a particular role in the management of pain in children with non-malignant life-limiting conditions in ACT/RCPCH groups III and IV (Chapter 2, Who needs it?, p. 17), because:

- this group is vulnerable to constipation and buprenorphine may carry less of a risk than other strong opioids;
- pain in this group is often relatively mild so that step 2 therapy is sufficient;
- a transdermal formulation is ideal since patients in this group are often gastrostomy or occasionally nasogastrically fed.

*But* even small doses of buprenorphine have been associated anecdotally with nausea and vomiting and even respiratory depression.

# When to move to step 3

Step 2 is insufficient if:
- codeine is needed regularly, or more than 3 times daily;
- breakthrough pain is occurring more than once or twice a day despite regular tramadol or buprenorphine;
- the adverse effects of drugs on step 2 are such that the burden outweighs their benefit.

In contrast with moving from step 1 to step 2, there is rarely a role for step 2 and step 3 opioids to be given concurrently. Minor opioids on step 2 should usually all be discontinued as soon as major opioids are commenced, as minor opioids do not induce adequate tolerance to the adverse effects of major opioids. Exceptions to this rule include:
- a small dose of oral morphine may be used for breakthrough alongside regular tramadol (effective potency of tramadol greater than OME would suggest);
- a high dose transdermal buprenorphine patch is effectively a major opioid, and therefore major opioids may also be appropriate for breakthrough doses.

## Reference

**1** World Health Organization (1998). Guidelines for analgesic drug therapy. In *Cancer pain relief and palliative care in children*, pp. 24–8. WHO/IASP Geneva.

# Pain: step 3, major opioids

# Introduction

Drugs at step 3 are considered major opioids (or sometimes 'strong opioids' or 'opioids for severe pain'). The choice of drugs available on this step is greater than on any of the others. Opioids can be considered as:
- naturally occurring ('opiates' such as morphine, diamorphine (heroin));
- synthetic (fentanyl, buprenorphine);
- semisynthetic (hydromorphone, pethidine (meperidine)).

Whilst the mechanism of action of opioids is similar, they may have distinct properties with respect to:
- action at opioid receptor subtypes ($\mu_1$, $\mu_2$, $\delta$, $\kappa$);
- action at non-opioid receptors (NMDA, substance P, etc.);
- potency;
- adverse effects profile;
- cost;
- formulation;
- availability;
- metabolism.

All of these should be taken into consideration when selecting the appropriate opioid for the situation. There are some general guiding principles (see also Table 4.1).
- Oral morphine is the major opioid of choice for first-line treatment because:
  - the research base in adults is strong;
  - the research base in children is stronger than for other opioids;
  - it is usually well tolerated;
  - it is usually effective, irrespective of the cause for pain.
- Major opioids should never be prescribed prn unless there is also regular background major opioid analgesia. There is no need for the two major opioids to be of the same class.
- Major opioids should never be prescribed regularly without also making available 'breakthrough' or prn doses.
- The breakthrough dose should always be one-sixth of the total daily dose, when standardized to 'oral morphine equivalence' (see box).
- The phenomena of tolerance, dependence, and addiction are distinct and should not be confused.
  - Tolerance: shift in the dose–response curve such that a greater dose of the drug is required for the same effect. This refers equally to desirable and adverse effects.
  - Dependence: physical changes that occur, often at receptor level, during long-term treatment with a drug that mean it should not be discontinued abruptly.
  - Addiction: complex physical, psychosocial, and spiritual phenomenon in which the individual is unable to function without the drug.

The evidence base for major opioids in children's palliative medicine has been the subject of reviews and book chapters[1–3] and is expanding all the time.

## Prescribing major opioids

In prescribing major opioids appropriately, the following should be taken into consideration.[1]

- Which drug?
- At what dose?
- By what route?

### Oral morphine equivalence (OME)

- OME is the observation that the potency of major opioids can be described in terms of each other by comparison with oral morphine (the 'standard unit' of opioid potency)
  - For example, oral diamorphine is approximately 1.5 times as potent as oral morphine, while oral hydromorphine is between 5 and 7.5 times the potency of oral morphine. Thus, the OME of oral diamorphine is 1.5, while that of oral hydromorphone would be between 5 and 7.5
- OME has largely been extrapolated from data in adults, but in practice seems to work well in children
- For most major opioids, bioavailability via iv, sc, transcutaneous, or transmucosal routes is considered to be twice that of oral bioavailability. Thus, the OME of diamorphine buccally is 3 ($2 \times 1.5$)

# Incomplete cross-tolerance

- Tolerance to different effects of a medication can develop at different rates in a single individual.
  - Tolerance to the analgesic effects of morphine occurs very slowly.
  - Tolerance to drowsiness develops within 2 or 3 days.
  - Tolerance to constipation does not develop at all.
- This is also true for different opioids, particularly those of different classes.
- Tolerance to analgesia may occur more slowly than tolerance to adverse effects.
- This means that changing to a different major opioid ('rotation' or 'substitution') can provide relief from some adverse effects (such as neuroexcitability) by allowing a reduction in OME opioid dose with no loss of analgesia.

# Morphine

Oral morphine is the major opioid of choice in palliative medicine. It is the archetypal major opioid.

## Strengths

- Powerfully analgesic in most pain.
- Usually well tolerated.
- Tolerance to its analgesic effects develops slowly and is easily managed by increasing the dose.
- Tolerance to some adverse effects develops quickly (especially drowsiness, which typically resolves within 48 hours of commencing morphine, with no modification in the dose).
- Evidence base in adult palliative medicine is excellent and in children very good.
- Available in slow- and immediate-release oral formulations as well as parenteral ones.

## Weaknesses

- Constipation: tolerance does not develop to constipation, and in most cases laxatives should be automatically co-prescribed. These should combine a stimulant with a softener such as co-danthrusate. (▶ Lactulose is neither and is not appropriate.)
- Respiratory depression: much feared but extremely rare.
- Fears of addiction: the risk is slight but the fears are real, and should be anticipated and pre-emptively addressed.
- Can be associated by child and/or family with 'terminal phase' and accelerated progress towards death.

# Alternative, non-morphine opioids

Use of non-morphine opioids in palliative care is a specialist skill and advice should be sought from the paediatric (or, if there is none, adult) palliative medicine team.

### Diamorphine
- OME 1.5.
- Formulations: parenteral, oral, buccal.
- Advantages over morphine: more highly soluble so can be given buccally and high doses can be dissolved in relatively small volumes.
- Disadvantages: as diamorphine rapidly cleaved to morphine after administration. Not suitable for rotation/substitution.
- Evidence base: as for morphine.

### Fentanyl
- OME 150.
- Available formulations: transdermal patch, parenteral, transmucosal (immediate release).
- Advantages over morphine:
  - complementary receptor profile; so works well alongside morphine breakthrough
  - available as a 72 hourly transdermal patch;
  - probably less constipating;
  - of a different class so suitable for opioid rotation/substitution.
- Disadvantages:
  - patches unsuitable for titration phase.
- Evidence base in children: good.
- Evidence base in adults: very good.

### Buprenorphine
- OME 60.
- Available formulations: transdermal patch, sublingual.
- Advantages over morphine:
  - available as a transdermal patch;
  - probably less constipating;
  - patch doses encompass steps 2 and 3 so can replace codeine;
  - of a different class so suitable for opioid rotation/substitution.
- Disadvantages: incidence of poor tolerability (nausea, vomiting, respiratory depression) higher than morphine, more difficult to reverse in overdosage as partial agonist.
- Evidence base in children: poor in palliative medicine; adequate in acute pain.
- Evidence base in adults: good.

### Methadone
- OME variable.
- Available formulations: oral, parenteral.
- Advantages over morphine:
  - probably has additional non-opioid effects (particularly NMDA blockade, giving adjuvant effect in neuropathic pain and potentially in bone pain);
  - different class from morphine so suitable for rotation/substitution.

- Disadvantages:
  - difficult to calculate conversion as OME variable depending on dose;
  - distributes to body fat, which becomes saturated, so theoretical risk of sudden fatal increase in serum concentration with no change in administered dose;
- Evidence base in children: many case series, some in palliative medicine.
- Evidence base in adults: very good.

## Hydromorphone

- OME 5–7.5.
- Available formulations: oral, parenteral.
- Advantages over morphine:
  - few in UK; in countries without access to diamorphine, provides alternative solution for dissolving high doses;
  - structurally similar to morphine, but probably different enough for effective rotation/substitution.
- Disadvantages:
  - slightly more expensive in most places.
- Evidence base in children: good, though most not in palliative medicine.
- Evidence base in adults: very good.

# At what dose and by what route?

The dose and route should be selected on the basis of the phase of management. There are three phases of opioid prescription:[1]

- initiation;
- titration;
- maintenance.

### Initiation

An appropriate starting dose can be arrived at by:
- Calculating on basis of weight (1mg/kg/24h OME) or
- Converting from existing opioid requirements on basis of OME (i.e. opioid rotation/substitution—see Chapter 7, Alternative, non-morphine opioids, p. 70).

For all prescriptions it is imperative to ensure:
- use of regular immediate release preparation initially;
- correct prescription of regular and breakthrough (see Table 4.1). (breakthrough dose should be one-sixth of total daily dose OME, given at least 4 hourly as needed);
- child and family know that breakthrough is available quickly when needed.

### Titration

The need for major opioid analgesia is matched against the intensity of pain over a period of days by:
- review of need for breakthrough over 48 hour period;
- recalculation of regular dose by adding to it the total daily requirements of breakthrough;
- recalculation of breakthrough so that it remains same proportion (one-sixth) of total;
- repeated review after 48 hours.

### Maintenance

Once pain has been matched by analgesia such that changes to the dose have become infrequent, convenience can be improved by switching to a long-acting formulation such as:
- slow-release morphine;
- transdermal patch (fentanyl, buprenorphine);
- syringe-driver (diamorphine, fentanyl).

▶ Even during the maintenance phase, breakthrough doses of an immediate-release formulation (ideally oral, e.g. morphine, methadone) should continue to be made available in the same proportion, i.e. one-sixth of the total daily dose OME.

## References

**1** Drake, R. and Hain, R. (2006). Pain—pharmacological management. In *Oxford textbook of palliative care for children* (ed. A. Goldman, R. Hain, and S. Liben), pp. 304–31 (particularly pp. 304–8). Oxford University Press, Oxford.

**2** Galloway, K.S. and Yaster, M. (2000). Pain and symptom control in terminally ill children. *Pediatr. Clin. North Am.* **47** (3), 711–46.

**3** Hewitt, M., Goldman, A., Collins, G.S., Childs, M., and Hain, R. (2008). Opioid use in palliative care of children and young people with cancer. *J. Pediatr.* **152**, 39–44.

# Adjuvants

# Introduction

- An adjuvant is not analgesic, but is capable of relieving pain in certain specific pain situations. Selection of an appropriate adjuvant is a key element of a rational and evidence-based approach to management of pain in children. It depends on diagnosis of the type of pain (see Diagnosis of pain, p. 78).
- Choice of an adjuvant is on the basis of the nature of pain, rather than its intensity. Suitable adjuvants should be considered at all three steps of the WHO pain ladder.

Adjuvants are more specific, but not necessarily more potent, than analgesics. For example:

  - amitriptyline is more specific to neuropathic pain than morphine **and**
  - neuropathic pain is less likely to be sensitive to morphine than other forms of pain **but**
  - the effectiveness of morphine is such that it is probably more likely to produce a beneficial effect than amitriptyline, even in neuropathic pain.

- Classic examples of adjuvants are anticonvulsants and antidepressants for relief of neuropathic pain.
- NSAIDs are usually considered adjuvants for bone pain but are in fact analgesic in their own right.

# Diagnosis of pain

Selection of a suitable adjuvant depends critically on recognizing the nature of the pain syndrome to be treated. A systematic approach to evaluation of pain, including its history, physical signs, and where necessary investigation, is essential (see Chapter 5). The box gives a useful mnemonic for taking a pain history.

There are many different ways to classify pain. For the purposes of selecting adjuvant medications, the most useful is the following.

### Neuropathic pain
This is characterized by:
- disordered sensation (numbness, allodynia, dysaesthesia, hyperaesthesia);
- a plausible nerve distribution such as a dermatome or, in the case of sympathetic mediated pain, a vascular distribution.

Central or thalamic pain, resulting from direct damage to the thalamus, is a special example of neuropathic pain that may be difficult to identify and treat.

### Bone pain
Characteristically:
- focal, deep seated, intense;
- occurring in the context of conditions causing metastasis or osteopenia;
- where these are complicated by pathological fracture or joint dislocation, may present as incident pain.

### Muscle spasm or colic
Typically:
- intense but short-lived;
- occurs in children without the cognitive or verbal ability to identify its location;
- between painful episodes, child may be pain-free.

### Cerebral irritation
Typically:
- follows acute brain injury such as perinatal asphyxia or intracerebral bleed;
- caused by amplification of pain and anxiety;
- occurs in the neonatal period, but may also result from trauma, infection, or malignancy in older children.

**Incident pain** is breakthrough pain from an intermittent cause (e.g. fracture) rather than from inadequate background analgesia. It can be difficult to treat and specialist paediatric (or, if that is not available, adult) palliative medicine advice should be sought.

## PQRST mnemonic for taking an adequate pain history

Using this, it should be possible to make a diagnosis of the likely pain syndrome and select the appropriate adjuvant accordingly

- Precipitating and relieving factors
- Quality of the pain (i.e. neuropathic? bone pain? muscle spasm?)
- Radiation of pain
- Severity of pain (use appropriate pain assessment tool)
- Timing of pain

# Adjuvants for neuropathic pain

**Anticonvulsants** (especially carbamazepine and gabapentin). Since seizures and pain both result from undesirable firing of neurons, it is understandable that anticonvulsants are effective in neuropathic type pain.

**Antidepressants,** particularly amitriptyline. Generally speaking, the older tricyclic antidepressants such as amitriptyline are more effective in managing neuropathic pain than later ones or antidepressants such as fluoxetine, which are of a different class. Amitriptyline also has sedative and anticholinergic properties that may be of additional benefit in symptom control. By the same token, however, these may limit its use in some patients. The antineuropathic dose of amitriptyline is approximately a fifth the antidepressant dose. Its analgesic effects are often seen within a few days.

**Lidocaine patches** are believed to provide a local effect through transdermal absorption.[1] Experience with their use in children is limited, but anecdotal reports suggest they may be of particular value in pain caused by tissues of neurogenic origin such as neurofibromas, neuroblastoma, or Ewing's sarcoma, particularly where these are superficial. The patches should be applied directly over the painful lesion.

## NMDA antagonists

The *N*-methyl D-aspartate receptors are involved in neuronal plasticity, i.e. the accommodation of a neural system to ongoing or repeated pain. The NMDA antagonist class of medications can relieve neuropathic pain through interference with this mechanism.

*Methadone* is, in principle, an ideal agent for relief of neuropathic pain, since it combines the properties of major opioid and NMDA antagonist. There is accumulating evidence of its safety and effectiveness in children[2] and it is generally well tolerated. In adults, regular methadone can result in saturation of body fat in such a way that there is a sudden increase in serum levels after a few days of treatment. In most adult palliative care units, therefore, it is only commenced on inpatients. This has severely limited its usefulness in children, whose palliative care is usually delivered in the home. It is unclear whether this 'secondary peak phenomenon' occurs in children, but it seems prudent to restrict methadone use to breakthrough pain, or to the small number of children whose palliative care is to be managed in an inpatient unit.

*Ketamine* The pain-relieving effects of ketamine can occur in doses much lower than those used for anaesthesia. Ketamine has long been used in children and its safety profile is well known. It is also known to result in frightening alterations in perception, particularly auditory hallucinations, and for that reason should be used with caution in children. A benefit of ketamine is that its oral bioavailability is very high so that it can be given enterally.

**Steroids** Because of their protean effects, steroids can be adjuvants for a wide range of pain conditions. Where nerve pain is caused by pressure (e.g. due to tumour) steroids can reduce oedema temporarily and help secure analgesia in the short term. The adverse effects of steroids mean that their use should usually be restricted to 2 or 3 days at a time, but this can be at high dose.

**Neurolytic procedures** (e.g. epidural anaesthetic, local regional anaesthesia, coeliac axis nerve block) can be highly effective. The necessity for a hospital admission and a needle means they are much less commonly used in paediatric palliative medicine than in the adult specialty. It can be difficult to provide analgesia without also impacting on motor function. Consultation with paediatric anaesthetic colleagues should be considered early, particularly when pain is focal and unrelieved by systemic measures.

# Adjuvants for bone pain

**NSAIDs** are not technically adjuvants since they have analgesic properties in their own right. They do, however, appear to have a specific role in managing bone pain. NSAIDs suppress production of inflammatory and pain mediators such as prostaglandins, thus reducing the sensation of pain and the cause of it. NSAIDs have a wide adverse effect profile, including gastrointestinal side effects, potential worsening of bronchospasm, and impacts on renal blood flow. In paediatric palliative care, the risk of severe adverse effects is usually outweighed by their potential benefit, but an individual judgement should clearly be made. Gastrointestinal side effects can be attenuated by judicious selection of formulation (e.g. enteric coated, or combined with gastric protectant misoprostol).

**Steroids** can reduce bone pain through reduction in inflammation and oedema around malignant microdeposits. They should be used with caution (see Chapter 8, Adjuvants for neuropathic pain, Steroids, pp. 80–81).

**Radiotherapy** For bone pain caused by metastatic deposits, radiotherapy can provide dramatic and long lasting relief from pain. This is particularly true of radiosensitive malignancies (e.g. leukaemias, Ewing's sarcoma), but good results can be obtained even in radioresistant disease (e.g. osteosarcoma). One visit to hospital for a single fraction of radiotherapy may be all that is necessary. Radiotherapy opinion should be sought whenever bone pain is caused by malignancy.

**Bisphosphonates** are pyrophosphate analogues that inhibit lytic activity of bone cortex by osteoclasts. Bisphosphonates have been used for some years[3] in adults with bone metastases. It is becoming clear[4] that they have a role in the much wider range of causes for bone pain seen in children. Evidence currently suggests that they are well tolerated by most children. Current guidelines suggest that iv pamidronate should be given at 3 monthly intervals, and that the initial dose should be given over 3 days as an inpatient. Subsequent doses can be given at home if the necessary nursing and medical support are available. Whilst their analgesic effects may be apparent within only a few weeks, patients should normally receive them for at least a year before a definitive assessment of their effectiveness can be made.

**Orthopaedic interventions** Where there is a specific bony injury or abnormality (such as hip dislocation, pathological fracture, or scoliosis), an orthopaedic opinion should always be sought. While, for many children, definitive corrective surgery may not be appropriate or even possible, there may be other interventions that can help. These may range from constructing pseudarthrosis to intra-articular injections of local anaesthetic and steroid.

**Neurolytic procedures** These can be effective, particularly if a single limb is the source for pain. They are uncomfortable and usually require hospital admission, both of which limit their usefulness in children (see Adjuvants for neuropathic pain, p. 80).

# Adjuvants for muscle spasm or intestinal colic

The term 'spasm' is used to mean at least three related but distinct phenomena:
- intermittent, intense, but short-lived contraction of muscles;
- chronic hypertonicity of muscles;
- seizure-like activity without changes in the EEG.

All three may occur in a single patient, particularly those in ACT/RCPCH groups III and IV.
- Seizure-like spasms may not be painful or distressing. Overtreatment may result in unnecessary adverse effects.
- Management of chronic muscle spasm should be in close collaboration with colleagues in neurodisability, community paediatrics, and paediatric neurology. Associated pain may be due to joint deformity and contractures rather than to muscle spasm itself.
- Acute muscle spasm is characterized by pain that is:
  - severe;
  - short-lived;
  - intermittent.

The main drug interventions available are:

## Benzodiazepines
- Buccal midazolam is rapidly absorbed and short acting. It can be administered by parents when acute muscle spasm occurs.
- If buccal midazolam is needed frequently, regular longer acting benzodiazepines (such as diazepam or lorazepam) may reduce the frequency of spasms.
- The metabolites of diazepam are active and long lasting but in children seem to be well tolerated.

## Antispasmodics: baclofen
- Baclofen can reduce the frequency and severity of painful muscle spasms.
- It tends to affect truncal muscle tone disproportionately (can adversely affect posture).
- It can be given orally, parenterally, or via intrathecal pump with good effect. (This requires input from specialist centres in Nottingham or Bristol.)
- Baclofen can reduce the seizure threshold and complicate management of fits.

## Other antispasmodics
There are numerous other antispasmodics available through specialist paediatric neurology services, including tizanidine, dantrolene, and cyclobenzaprine.

## Botulinum toxin
- Given by local injection into muscle.
- Effects last several weeks.

- Can give an indication of potential benefit from orthopaedic interventions, e.g. tenotomy.
- Effects can accumulate, leading to systemic neurological problems.
- Requires specialist orthopaedic or neurodisability involvement.

### Need for team working

In managing symptomatic muscle spasm, it is important to collaborate closely with colleagues coordinating seizure medication because:

- some antispasmodics can change seizure threshold and therefore complicate anticonvulsant management;
- some anticonvulsants are also effective antispasmodics, reducing the risk of unnecessary polypharmacy;
- specialist neurology interventions may be effective where palliative care ones have failed (e.g. tizanidine, botulinum toxin).

# Adjuvants for cerebral irritation

Cerebral irritation is a form of 'total' pain. It comprises:
- pain from physical causes such as cerebral oedema, cerebral haemorrhage;
- anxiety, exacerbated by inability to process neurological stimuli and understand their context;
- temporal disorientation and disruption of the sleep/wake cycle;
- reflected anxiety from exhausted and sleep-deprived carers.

Cerebral irritation is caused by acute inflammation.
- Following hypoxic ischaemic encephalopathy in the neonatal period, treatment should continue for 3–6 months and gradually give way to conventional management of the effects of residual neurological deficit.
- Following acute cerebral trauma or infection, treatment should continue in a similar way.
- Where caused by malignant disease, treatment should continue until death unless some other intervention such as palliative chemotherapy or radiotherapy intervenes.
- Phenobarbital, benzodiazepines, and opioids should be weaned gradually in order to avoid rebound symptoms.

Suitable adjuvants include the following.
- Phenobarbital. An effective soporific and anxiolytic. It is also a useful anticonvulsant, though its long-term use is restricted by adverse effects. Phenobarbital can be given orally or via parenteral infusion. Although phenobarbital can be given subcutaneously, it cannot be combined with most other medications. It requires a dedicated syringe driver, which may be unacceptable to some families.
- Benzodiazepines. A combination of:
  - long acting benzodiazepine (e.g. lorazepam, diazepam);
  - immediate and short acting (e.g. buccal midazolam) for 'breakthrough' cerebral irritation.
- Opioids. Whilst most children with cerebral irritation cannot express that they are in pain, it seems a reasonable assumption since the causes of cerebral irritation are also causes for pain (acute brain injury, leptomeningeal metastatic spread, acute inflammation).

## References

**1** Nayak, S. and Cunliffe, M. (2008). Lidocaine 5% patch for localized chronic neuropathic pain in adolescents: report of five cases. *Paediatr. Anaesth.* **18** (6), 554–8.

**2** Davies, D., DeVlaming, D., and Haines, C. (2008). Methadone analgesia for children with advanced cancer. *Pediatr. Blood Cancer* **51** (3), 393–7.

**3** Colvin, L. and Fallon, M. (2008). Challenges in cancer pain management—bone pain. *Eur. J. Cancer* **44** (8), 1083–90.

**4** Gonzalez, E., Pavia, C., Ros, J., Villaronga, M., Valls, C., and Escola, J. (2001). Efficacy of low dose schedule pamidronate infusion in children with osteogenesis imperfecta. *J. Pediatr. Endocrinol. Metab.* **14** (5), 529–33.

# Nausea and vomiting

# Introduction

The management of nausea and vomiting requires an understanding of the probable mechanism and logical consideration of drug selection. But it also requires an approach that is individualized to the emotional and psychological needs of the child and family.

The evolutionary purpose of vomiting is to expel ingested toxins before they can do damage. Vomiting gives the body several opportunities to do this.

- Even the smell or sight of something nauseous can evoke a powerful emetic response (anticipatory nausea).
- Once a toxin is ingested, emesis can be initiated in the gastrointestinal tract, the liver, or the brain.
- It is mediated by a series of receptors and neurochemicals, modified (and often amplified) by emotional and psychological input from higher cortical centres, coordinated by a specialized centre of the brain, and finally effected via the vagus nerve.

Palliative medicine concerns patients in whom:
- anxiety levels are often high;
- there may be a multiplicity of physical factors;

Effective management of the symptom requires attention to all dimensions. This involves the following.

- It is important to explore the expectations of the patient and family before embarking on treatment.
- It is also important to be realistic about what can be achieved.
- Even with optimal pharmacological and psychological support, it is not always possible to abolish nausea and vomiting entirely.
- For most patients, reducing the frequency of vomiting to once or twice a day may be enough.
- As always, there is a need to balance the likely impact of antiemetic therapy against the potential adverse effects. The balance of burden and benefit for individual families needs to be established before embarking on treatment.

# Pathophysiology: receptors

Most research in children has been in nausea and vomiting associated with chemotherapy.[1,2] Nausea and vomiting is known to be a significant symptom among children needing palliative care, particularly in cancer.[3–5] A rational approach in adults[6] has been proposed, but never validated in children.

The mechanism of the physiological basis of nausea and vomiting is essentially an interaction of neurochemicals with receptors. Each of the organs primarily involved in nausea and vomiting is associated with a group of receptors. Most antiemetics work by blocking one or more of the receptors. No antiemetic blocks all receptors.

Most is known about 6 antiemetic receptors:

- $D_2$ dopamine receptor. Found in gastrointestinal tract and centrally. Blocked by metoclopromide and haloperidol.
- $H_1$ histamine receptor. Associated with intracranial and vestibular causes, blocked, along with ACh, by cyclizine.
- Acetylcholine associated with vestibular causes, and with vagal nerve. Hyoscine is a pure acetylcholine blocker.
- $5HT_2$ serotonin receptor. Associated with the bowel wall; blocked, among other things, by levomepromazine.
- $5HT_3$. Associated with bowel wall; blocked by ondansetron and similar drugs.
- $5HT_4$. Associated with bowel wall; blocked by high dose metoclopromide.

A further class of receptors has recently been identifed, with three sub-types associated with the bowel mucosa. They are neurokinin receptors $NK_1$, $NK_2$, and $NK_3$. This further opens up the possibilities for pharmacological intervention using antagonists. To date, only one neurokinin antagonist has been fully developed. Aprepitant, a pure $NK_1$ antagonist, has been studied in adults and appears to be well tolerated with good effect.[7]

## Organs

Four organs are particularly involved in nausea and vomiting: the gastrointestinal tract; the bloodstream; the liver; and the brain. In considering a rational approach to managing nausea and vomiting, it is first necessary to decide which of these is or are the main cause(s).

### Gastrointestinal

- Mucosal damage:
  - chemotherapy ($D_2$, $5HT_3$);
  - radiotherapy ($5HT_{3,4}$);
  - obstruction.
- Mechanical:
  - obstruction;
  - reflux.

### Blood (toxins)

- Medication ($D_2$).
- Infection ($5HT_2$).
- Constipation ($5HT_{3,4}$).

*Liver damage*
- Focal deposits (physical effect).
- Diffuse disease ($5HT_4$).

*Brain*
- Vestibular:
  - vertigo (ACh);
  - travel sickness ($H_1$).
- Raised intracranial pressure:
  - tumour ($H_1$);
  - oedema.
- Psychological:
  - anticipation;
  - anxiety (benzodiazepine receptors).

▶ The motor pattern that constitutes the act of vomiting is generated in a specialized part of the brain, the vomiting centre (also known as the emetic pattern generator), and effected via the vagus nerve (ACh).

# Pathophysiology: non-receptor mechanisms

Drug–receptor interactions are not the only links in the chain of causality for nausea and vomiting. It may be possible to modify other factors.

## Physical factors

Can contribute to:
- raised intracranial pressure (e.g. brain tumour, cerebral oedema);
- liver damage (e.g. metastatic cancer, particularly where the liver capsule is stretched);
- gastrointestinal obstruction;
- reflux.

## Psychological factors

There is often a close association between anxiety and nausea and vomiting. Two common situations are the following.

### Anticipation

Commonly occurs when there is a strong association between an emetogenic stimulus such as chemotherapy and a specific environment such as oncology outpatients, in which sight, sound, and especially smell combine to reinforce the association over succeeding visits.

The association between environment, event, and emesis needs to be broken. This can be done using:
- play or psychotherapy;
- hypnotherapy;
- medications that attenuate the experience of anxiety, particularly nabilone (mildly euphoric derivative of marijuana with sedative and antiemetic properties) and benzodiazepines;
- complementary therapies.

### Generalized anxiety

The above measures may be used. Benzodiazepines are anxiolytic, whereas soporifics (e.g. chloral hydrate, levomepromazine) are not.
- Midazolam. Can be given parenterally or buccally.
  - Advantage: rapid onset, short acting, amnestic.
  - Disadvantages: may be so short acting that it does not encompass whole stressful episode.
- Lorazepam. May be given orally, parenterally, or sublingually.
  - Advantages: longer acting, can be rapid onset if given sublingually.
  - Disadvantages: long duration of action may not always be desirable.
- Diazepam. Can be given orally or parenterally or rectally.
  - Advantages: longer acting.
  - Disadvantages: may be too long acting.

In general, as with most medications for managing psychological aspects of illness, they should not be prescribed alone but in association with appropriate non-drug techniques.

# Management

Rational drug management of nausea and vomiting depends on:
- inferring or demonstrating what mechanisms are at work;
- understanding what receptors are likely to be involved;
- understanding what non-receptor mechanisms are likely to be involved.

## Before embarking on medications

- Invasive investigations may not be justified in children close to death as a diagnosis and rational management plan is usually possible without it.
- It is often not possible to abolish nausea and vomiting entirely, and this needs to be made clear from the outset, along with the assurance that significant improvement is very likely.
- Establish with child and family what their goals are for managing the problem.
- Consider non-physical contributions to the symptom, and also physical contributions that can be managed in a non-pharmacological way (see Chapter 9, Pathophysiology: non-receptor mechanisms, p. 94).

## Medications

Pharmacologically, a logical approach is as follows.
- Choose a rational first-line drug (i.e. one likely to block the appropriate receptors).
- Review the effectiveness of this approach.
- If this fails, choose a rational second-line drug. This can be one of three things:
  - an alternative drug, because in the meantime an alternative explanation for the problem has become clear;
  - a complementary drug, i.e. one that blocks some of the receptors that were not blocked by your first choice;
  - an alternative antiemetic that blocks a much wider range of receptors. Phenothiazines, and in particular levomepromazine, are 'broad spectrum' antiemetics and can be useful second-line drugs.

Table 9.1 shows the receptor antagonist properties of common antiemetics. On the basis of an understanding of those receptor properties, and of the likely mechanism of nausea and vomiting in your patient, it should be possible to derive a logical approach.

### Steroids

Long-term steroids should be avoided in paediatric palliative medicine as their benefits are quickly outweighed by their adverse effects. Short courses of steroids may, however, be helpful adjuvants in managing nausea and vomiting. Steroids probably do not work directly through a drug–receptor interaction, but by:
- reducing oedema, particularly in the brain (e.g. brain tumour) or in the liver (e.g. infection or metastatic disease);
- reducing inflammation; by moderating the inflammatory response, steroids can reduce the amount of cell damage and release of mediators of emesis.

**Table 9.1** Some causes of nausea and vomiting and appropriate anti-emetics for treating them

| Likely cause | Example | Antiemetic (receptor) |
|---|---|---|
| Vestibular | Vertigo or travel sickness | Hyoscine (ACh) or cyclizine (ACh, $H_1$) |
| Toxins | Medications, particularly chemotherapy | Metoclopramide, haloperidol ($D_2$) |
| | Infections (endotoxins) | Ondansetron, etc. ($5HT_3$) |
| | Constipation | Metoclopramide ($5HT_4$) |
| Gastrointestinal damage | Chemotherapy | Metoclopramide ($D_2$, $5HT_4$) |
| | | Ondansetron, etc. ($5HT_3$) |
| | | Steroids (inflammation) |
| Liver damage | Focal deposits | Metoclopramide ($5HT_4$) |
| | Diffuse disease | Steroids (inflammation) |
| Psychological | Anticipation and anxiety | Non-physical |
| | | Benzodiazepine receptors |
| | | Nabilone |
| Raised intracranial pressure | Tumour | Cyclizine ($H_1$) |
| | Oedema | Steroids (oedema) |

# Reflux

In children with life-limiting conditions that are non-malignant, reflux is an important differential diagnosis from true nausea and vomiting. The main causes are:
- lax gastro-oesophegeal sphincter caused by muscle incoordination;
- painful and dangerous acid reflux;
- loss of normal reflex bowel motility, causing overdistension, particularly by continuous feeds.

Each of these factors can be managed rationally.
- Lax gastro-oesophageal sphincter:
  - $D_2$ blockers, e.g. metoclopramide.
- Painful and dangerous acid reflux:
  - $H_2$ blockers, e.g. ranitidine;
  - proton blockers, e.g. omeprazole;
  - Gaviscon®.
- Loss of normal reflex bowel motility:
  - change feed timings to avoid overfull stomach;
  - dopamine blockers.

# Rational approach to antiemesis

The box and Fig. 9.1 summarize a rational approach to the treatment of nausea and vomiting.

## Summary of antiemetic approaches

- All children:
  - explain, reassure, and modify diet to ensure it consists of frequent, low-volume, attractive foods
  - treat anxiety (see Chapter 14)
- Possible iatrogenic causes?
  - review drug list and stop non-essential emetogenic drugs
- Non-pharmacological management?
  - anxiety reduction (see Chapter 14)
- Features of gastritis or oesophagitis (pain, indigestion, flatulence, blood in vomit)?
  - stop NSAIDs and steroids if possible
  - use omeprazole or ranitidine
  - if not available try magnesium trisilicate (although not well tolerated in children)
- Features of gastric stasis or compression (e.g. known abdominal tumour or abdominal organomegaly)?
  - try gastric motility stimulant (domperidone or metoclopramide)
- Related to movement?
  - rule out iatrogenic cause
  - start vestibular-active drug such as cyclizine or hyoscine hydrobromide
- Related to toxic or systemic causes (e.g. infections, advanced tumours, renal or hepatic failure)?
  - treat underlying cause where possible
  - use drugs active on CNS receptors, such as promazine, haloperidol, cyclizine
- Features of raised intracranial pressure?
  - consider radiotherapy or shunt
  - if not appropriate, cyclizine is drug of choice.
  - consider steroids but see cautions in Chapter 13
- Above suggestions not working or is sedation indicated?
  - try levomepromazine (if available)

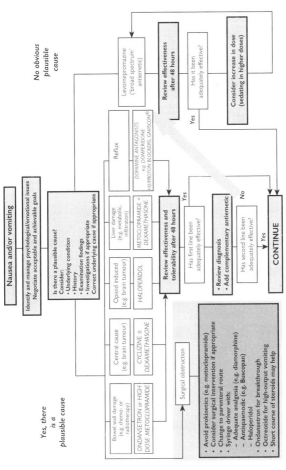

**Fig. 9.1** A flow chart outlining a rational approach to antiemesis.

## Summary

- Evaluate, negotiate, and investigate only as appropriate for the individual child in the individual family
- Choose rational first-line drug, based on understanding of likely aetiology and of antiemetic pharmacology
- Review effectiveness and tolerability
- If ineffective, choose rational alternative, complement, or switch to broad spectrum antiemetic such as levomepromazine, which blocks many receptors
- Always consider psychosocial and emotional components and address these using non-drug and drug interventions

# References

**1** Antonarakis, E.S., Evans, J.L., Heard, G.F., Noonan, L.M., Pizer, L., and Hain, R. (2004). Prophylaxis of acute chemotherapy-induced nausea and vomiting in children with cancer: What is the evidence? *Pediatr. Blood Cancer* **43** (6), 651–8.

**2** Antonarakis, E.S. and Hain, R. (2004). Nausea and vomiting associated with cancer chemotherapy: drug management in theory and in practice. *Arch. Dis. Child.* **89** (9), 877–80.

**3** Goldman, A., Hewitt, M., Collins, G.S., Childs, M., and Hain, R. (2006). Symptoms in children/ young people with progressive malignant disease: United Kingdom Children's Cancer Study Group/Paediatric Oncology Nurses Forum survey. *Pediatrics* **117** (6), e1179–86.

**4** Hongo, T., Watanabe, C., Okada, S., Inoue, N., Yajima, S., Fujii, Y., *et al.* (2003). Analysis of the circumstances at the end of life in children with cancer: symptoms, suffering and acceptance. *Pediatr. Int.* **45** (1), 60–4.

**5** Wolfe, J., Grier, H.E., Klar, N., Levin, S.B., Ellenbogen, J.M., Salem-Schatz, S., *et al.* (2000. Symptoms and suffering at the end of life in children with cancer [see comments]. *N. Engl. J. Med.* **342** (5), 326–33.

**6** Twycross, R. and Back, I. (1998). Nausea and vomiting in advanced cancer. *Eur. J. Palliative Care* **5** (2), 39–45.

**7** Warr, D.G., Hesketh, P.J., Gralla, R.J., Muss, H.B., Herrstedt, J., Eisenberg, P.D., *et al.* (2005). Efficacy and tolerability of aprepitant for the prevention of chemotherapy-induced nausea and vomiting in patients with breast cancer after moderately emetogenic chemotherapy. *J. Clin. Oncol.* **23** (12), 2822–30.

# Gastrointestinal symptoms

# Constipation

**Definition** The number of times a child normally opens their bowels is very variable and age-dependent. A normal breast fed baby may do so up to 10 times day or only once or twice a week. Aged 2–3 years the mean is 2 times a day and above this age between 3 times a day to 3 times a week. It is best in paediatrics to think of alteration in bowel habits as a way of detecting constipation.

## General points

- All children with constipation need a structured assessment, with formal medical, drug, dietary, and social history. Then examination of the abdomen with rectal examination if appropriate. Once cause is established then a rational choice of medication should be used.
- Rectal examination should only ever be done by experienced physicians or nurses after appropriate explanation to the patient and carers. Children often find this distressing, particularly if they have an anal tear or have had repeated examinations.
- Although diet is important in the management of constipation, many of the children with special needs struggle to chew food or even swallow. Food often has to be pureed or given as feeds via gastrostomies or nasogastric tubes, after having been specially designed and calculated for them by dietitians.
- Good communication with the carers is essential as they know their child's habits, and they may have misconceptions about defecation and the use of laxatives.

## Cause

- Inactivity: due to illness or treatment. The child having chemotherapy in bed or the wheelchair bound child with a neurodegenerative disorder.
- Neurological: damage to nerve pathways and musculature secondary to neurodegenerative disease.
- Specific illness: cystic fibrosis.
- Metabolic: hypercalcaemia or hypokalaemia.
- Dehydration.
- Decreased food intake or abnormal feeding patterns.
- Fear of opening bowels: due to constipation pain or lack of privacy.
- Anal tears: from passing hard stools.
- Social: related to not using toilets they are not used to or fear of bothering carers.
- Drugs:
  - opioids;
  - anticholinergics such as hyoscine;
  - anticonvulsants;
  - $5HT_3$ antagonists;
  - NSAIDs;
  - tricyclic antidepressants;
  - iron;
  - chemotherapy drugs such as vincristine;
  - benzodiazepines;
  - $H_2$ receptor antagonists;
  - proton pump inhibitors.

# Management of constipation

## Diagnosis
- Correct diagnosis of the type of constipation.
- Assess possibility of impaction or overflow presenting as diarrhoea or faecal soiling.

## Treatment
Know which drugs are used to treat the different types of constipation (see Table 10.1).
- Step 1. Start with an osmotic laxative building up the dose slowly over a week.
- Step 2. If no improvement, add a stimulant laxative such as senna or change to co-danthramer (caution with licence).
- If the child is starting an opioid then ignore step 1 and go straight to step 2.
- Step 3. If constipation persists then perform rectal examination:
  - if stool hard, use lubricant suppository such as glycerin;
  - if stool soft, use stimulant suppository such as bisacodyl;
  - if rectum empty, use bisacodyl suppository to bring stool down or high phosphate enema.
- Step 4. If severely constipated use Micralax® or phosphate enema, or if you have time, paediatric Movicol® (see box).
- If anal fissure apparent, or manual removal required, then use a topical anaesthetic gel, e.g. lidocaine ointment, or discuss possibility of a short general anaesthetic.

### Macrogol: Movicol® Paediatric Plain
- An iso-osmotic laxative
- Flavour- and sweetener-free
- Requires 60mL of water per sachet
- Licensed for children > 1 year
- Very effective, particularly for impaction:
  - for 1–5 year old child use up to 8 sachets;
  - for 5–12 year old child, use up to 12 sachets

## Novel approaches
- Oral naloxone has been used in adult care to alleviate opioid-induced constipation.[2]
- Erythromycin has a side effect of increased bowel motility and this has been used successfully in resistant cases.[3]
- Prokinetic drugs such as metoclopramide or domperidone have all been tried with varying success.

**Table 10.1** Drugs used to treat constipation*

| Type/drugs | Onset speed | Mechanism | Comment |
|---|---|---|---|
| Lubricant, e.g. paraffin or glycerin suppositories | 1–3 days | Penetrates stools & softens; glycerin also has osmotic effect | Paraffin: taste & risk of inhalation, particularly in children with gastro-oesophageal reflux, limit use. No longer recommended for internal use. Glycerine: suppository effective for hard stool |
| Bulk-forming, e.g. ispaghula | 2–4 days | Acts as stool normalizer | Very limited use in paediatric palliative care |
| Osmotic | 1–4 days | Exerts osmotic influence in small bowel and so retains water in lumen | |
| Surfactant, e.g. sodium docusate or poloxamer | po: 1–3 days<br>pr: 20 min | Acts as detergent & increases water penetration into stool; also acts as stimulant laxative | Docusate can be used by itself. Poloxamer is combined to make co-danthramer. Other similar compounds found in mini-enemas |
| Saline, e.g. magnesium hydroxide or sulphate, sodium sulphate | 1–6 hours | Osmotic effect in all of gut. Increases water secretion and stimulates peristalsis | Not used much in very ill children because of strong purgative action. Very effective in difficult cases. Repeated use inappropriate; can cause biochemical imbalance |
| Anthraquinones, e.g. senna and danthron<br><br>Diphenylmethane, e.g. bisacodyl and sodium picosulphate | po: 6–12 hours<br><br>pr: 15–60 min | Directly stimulates myenteric plexus | Senna commonly used in liquid form; combines well with lactulose. Dantron is used in combinations, e.g. co-danthramer. Bisacodyl can be given po or pr. Particularly useful in its suppository form. Reserve sodium picosulphate for most difficult cases |

* Modified from Jassal, S,. (2007). *Basic symptom control in paediatric palliative care, the Rainbows Children's Hospice guidelines*, 7th edn. Rainbows Children's Hospice, Loughborough.

# Anorexia

**Definition** Anorexia can be thought of as poor appetite or loss of desire to eat. It is very common in all types of paediatric terminal conditions. It causes great distress to families as it goes against the primal instinct to feed children.

## Causes
- Pain: either generalized or specific to eating.
- Anxiety.
- Depression.
- Nausea or vomiting.
- Dyspepsia.
- Thrush in the mouth or oesophagus.
- Constipation.
- Drugs: including chemotherapy agents.
- Radiotherapy.
- Certain smells.
- Food presentation.
- Altered tastes.
- Disease process.

## Management
- Look at the possible causes and treat appropriately.
- Reassure parents that an inactive child will have a reduced requirement for food.
- Alter food:
  - use smaller portions;
  - use smaller plates;
  - encourage more frequent meals;
  - allow parents to give their children fast foods;
  - be flexible with timings of meals;
  - make food less effort to eat—mash, soups. etc.
- Involve dietitian early.
- Use food supplements but remember they often do not taste good but can be made more palatable by serving cold.
- Anabolic steroids such as prednisolone or dexamethasone can be used in short 5–7 day bursts to increase appetite. Unfortunately, their side effects, particularly those of body distortion, severely limit their longer term use.
- Other medical stimulants of appetite include some antipsychotics and other psychoactive medications. Again, the adverse effects of these are often significant and they should be used with great caution in children. There is a risk of prescribing medications to a child in order to treat their parents' need to feed the child.

# Cachexia

**Definition** A condition associated with decrease in appetite with associated increase in metabolism of fat and lean body mass. It leads to damage to skeletal muscle (pale fibres more affected than red) causing profound lethargy and fatigue. There is major weight loss with associated alteration of body image which can be very distressing to the child and family.

## Causes
- Endogenous acute response to illness or injury.
- Thought to be metabolic.
- Leads to **cachexia/anorexia syndrome**.
- Linked with many chronic and end stage conditions.
- More common in solid tumour cancer than in haematological cancers.

## Management
- Manage the causes of anorexia.
- Although cachexia is not characterized by low calorie intake it is often associated with it, so it is always worth trying high calorie diets.
- Drugs: a number are being tried in adult palliative care but evidence of use in paediatrics is poor.
  - anabolic steroids;
  - human growth hormone;
  - testosterone;
  - appetite stimulants: megestrol;
  - NSAIDs;
  - cytokine antagonists;
  - nutritional supplements: omega-3 fatty acids.

# Hiccup

**Definition** Hiccups occur when there is involuntary contraction of the diaphragm resulting in sudden inspiration followed by abrupt closure of the glottis.

It is a common condition, but is more likely to become pathological in the palliative care setting. It is classified as persistent when lasting longer than 2 days or intractable if longer than 1 month.

## Causes
- Gastrointestinal:
  - GORD;
  - gastric distension;
  - diaphragmatic irritation.
- Phrenic nerve irritation.
- Biochemical:
  - uraemia;
  - hyponatraemia;
  - hypocalcaemia;
  - liver dysfunction.
- Stress and insomnia.
- Pyrexia.
- Infection.
- Intracranial lesion.
- Drugs:
  - corticosteroids;
  - antidepressants;
  - antibiotics;
  - analgesics including opioids.
- Many of the drugs used to treat hiccups can also induce them.

## Management[4–6]
- Gastric distension:
  - defoaming antiflatulent such as Asilone® or Maalox® Plus
  - prokinetic drug that tightens lower oesophageal sphincter such as metoclopramide;
  - peppermint water relaxes lower oesophageal sphincter to aid belching (do not use with metoclopramide).
- GORD:
  - metoclopramide;
  - $H_2$ antagonists;
  - proton pump inhibitors.
- Diaphragmatic irritation:
  - baclofen as a muscle relaxant;
  - chlorpromazine;
  - reports in adults of benefits with nifedipine and midazolam.
- Stimulation of pharynx (folk remedies):
  - swallowing crushed ice;
  - cold key down back;
  - shouting 'boo' to produce startle response.

- Stimulation of pharynx (medically based):
  - normal saline 2mL nebulized over 5min;
  - oropharyngeal stimulation with NG tube;
  - massage at junction of hard and soft palate with cotton bud;
  - forced retraction of tongue to induce gag reflex;
  - vagal stimulation through carotid massage or Valsalva manoeuvre.
- Central suppression of hiccup reflex:
  - metoclopramide;
  - chlorpromazine;
  - baclofen;
  - sodium valproate, phenytoin, or carbamazepine;
  - elevating $PaCO_2$ in the brainstem by breath holding or breathing in and out of a paper bag.

# Diarrhoea

**Definition** An increase in frequency or fluidity of bowel motions.

## Causes
- Gastroenteritis.
- HIV/AIDS most common palliative cause in the world.
- Faecal impaction.
- Malabsorption/diet.
- Pancreatic exocrine deficiency (cystic fibrosis).
- Drug-induced:
  - directly: NSAID;
  - indirectly: antibiotics.
- Post radiation/chemotherapy.
- Concurrent illness such as colitis.

## Management[7,8]
- Reassurance.
- Clear fluids.
- Electrolyte replacement.
- Stool cultures to look for infection.
- Herbal remedies such a live yoghurt.
- Drugs including:
  - codeine;
  - loperamide;
  - co-phenotrope.
- Specific antimicrobial, fungicidal, and antiparasitic treatment, particularly in HIV-related diarrhoea.
- Pancreatic enzyme replacement.

# Sialorrhoea

**Definition** A condition of loss of control of saliva, often seen as drooling with leakage of saliva from the mouth.

## Physiology

Sialorrhoea can be caused by three different factors:
- excessive production of saliva;
- inability to retain saliva in the mouth;
- difficulty in swallowing.

Excessive production is not a problem in itself unless accompanied by one or both of the other two factors.

## Symptoms
- Dermatitis around mouth, lips, and chin.
- Constant need to change bibs and clothing.
- Choking.
- Coughing.
- Aspiration pneumonia.
- Dysphagia.
- Breathing difficulties.
- Social stigma.[9]

## Causes
- Neurodegenerative disorders: 10% of all cases and up to half of all children with cerebral palsy.[10]
- Abnormalities of the mouth, jaw, or nasopharynx.
- Cancer affecting mouth.
- Dysphagia.
- Psychological.
- Drugs including:
  - cholinergic drugs;
  - neuroleptics.

## Management[11,12]

Saliva consists of two components, a thin watery secretion and a thick mucus. These are produced by different salivary glands. Treatment tends to affect these two components differently and can cause the paradoxical problem of reducing saliva production but producing thick mucus in the throat that is difficult to cough up.

Treatment requires a logical and pragmatic approach. Pharmacological treatments only work in 50% of cases and, even then, become less effective over time.
- Treat local factors:
  - dental hygiene;
  - dermatitis with mild steroids, antibiotics, moisturizers, or barrier creams;
  - sore gums and mouth ulcers with topical analgesics.
- Review medication, which may be exacerbating the problem.

### Scopolamine (hyoscine hydrobromide)
- Comes in various formulations but patch most useful, as it avoids first pass liver effect so smaller doses can be used.
- Put patch behind ear.
- Lasts 72h.
- Smaller doses can be given by occluding part of patch. In our unit we cut the patch, although this is out of licence.
- Side effects include: behavioural problems, constipation, cardiac arrythmia, urinary retention, flushing, nausea, giddiness and confusion, restlessness, and blurred vision.

### Glycopyrronium bromide
- Comes in oral formulation.
- Similar effectiveness and side effects to hyoscine.
- Tends to cause less central effects such as confusion.

### Tricyclic antidepressant
- The side effect of these drugs is dry mouth which is used to treat the sialorrhoea.
- Central effects may help the mood of the child.

### Botulinum toxin A[13]
- Injected into the parotid and submandibular glands.
- Should be done under ultrasound control as injection into other sites may lead to paralysis of critical muscles.
- Limited data on effectiveness.
- Only lasts 3–8 months (may get longer effect with repeated injections due to gland hypotrophy).

### Surgery[14]
- Three approaches: removing salivary glands, ligating salivary ducts, or sectioning nerve supply (denervation procedures reduce taste to anterior two-thirds of tongue).
- Poor success with all types of surgery.
- Current view is for duct ligation of parotid and submandibular glands.

## References

1 Hanson, S. and Bansal, N. (2006). The clinical effectiveness of Movicol in children with severe constipation: an outcome audit. *Paediatr. Nurs.* **18** (2), 24–8.

2 Tofil, N.M., Benner, K.W., Faro, S.J., and Winkler, M.K. (2006). The use of enteral naloxone to treat opioid-induced constipation in a pediatric intensive care unit. *Pediatr. Crit. Care Med.* **7** (3), 252–4.

3 Bellomo-Brandao, M.A., Collares, E.F., and da-Costa-Pinto, E.A. (2003). Use of erythromycin for the treatment of severe chronic constipation in children. *Braz. J. Med. Biol. Res,* **36** (10), 1391–6.

4 Friedman, N.L. (1996). Hiccups: a treatment review. *Pharmacotherapy* **16** (6), 986–95.

5 Lewis, J.H. (1985). Hiccups: causes and cures. *J. Clin. Gastroenterol.* **7** (6), 539–52.

6 Lipsky, M.S. (1986). Chronic hiccups. *Am. Fam. Physician* **34** (5), 173–7.

7 Cézard, J-P., Bellaiche, M., Viala, J., and Hugo, J-P. (2007). [Medication in infectious acute diarrhea in children]. *Arch. Pediatr.* **14** (Suppl. 3), S169–75.

8 Karan, S. (1979). Lomotil in diarrhoeal illnesses. *Arch. Dis. Child.* **54** (12), 984.

9 Van der Burg, J.J., *et al.* (2006). Drooling in children with cerebral palsy: effect of salivary flow reduction on daily life and care. *Dev. Med. Child Neurol.* **48** (2), 103–7.

10 Morales Chavez, M.C., Nualart Grollmus, Z.C., and Silvestre-Donat, F.J. (2008). Clinical prevalence of drooling in infant cerebral palsy. *Med. Oral Patol. Oral Cir. Bucal.* **13** (1), E22–6.

11 Tscheng, D.Z. (2002). Sialorrhea—therapeutic drug options. *Ann. Pharmacother.* **36** (11), 1785–90.

12 Jongerius, P.H., van Tiel, P., van Limbeek, J., Gabreëls, F.J.M., and Rotteveel, J.J. (2003). A systematic review for evidence of efficacy of anticholinergic drugs to treat drooling. *Arch. Dis. Child.* **88** (10), 911–14.

13 Reid, S.M., Johnstone, B.R., Westbury, C., Rawicki, B., and Reddihough, D.S. (2008). Randomized trial of botulinum toxin injections into the salivary glands to reduce drooling in children with neurological disorders. *Dev. Med. Child. Neurol.* **50** (2), 123–8.

14 Greensmith, A.L., Johnstone, B.R., Reid, S.M., Hazard, C.J., Johnson, H.M., and Reddihough, D.S. (2005). Prospective analysis of the outcome of surgical management of drooling in the pediatric population: a 10 year experience. *Plast. Reconstr. Surg.* **116** (5), 1233–42.

# Mouth care, feeding, and hydration

# Mouth care

## General points
- This is an often overlooked area of symptom management as doctors typically have little training in oral medicine.
- Pathology in the mouth can have a considerable effect on the child's ability to communicate and to eat.
- Maintenance of oral hygiene can often be done by parents, and this allows them to be actively involved in helping their child through actions that are perceived to be part of normal parenting.
- Successful management can considerably improve the quality of a child's life.
- Be aware that a high sugar diet (including medication) can lead to tooth decay.
- Correct management requires taking a good history, always looking inside the mouth, and basic clinical skills.

## Cause of mouth symptoms
- Poor oral hygiene.
- Oral candidiasis:
  - antibiotics;
  - corticosteroids;
  - general debility.
- Dry mouth:
  - mouth breathing;
  - dehydration;
  - oxygen that has not been humidified;
  - anxiety;
  - drugs: opioids, antihistamines, antimuscarinics, antidepressants, diuretics;
  - radiotherapy;
  - stomatitis secondary to neutropenia;
  - direct damage to salivary glands from tumour infiltration or radiotherapy;
  - hypercalcaemia or hyperglycaemia.
- Mouth ulcers:
  - infection;
  - traumatic;
  - aphthous.
- Bleeding gums:
  - poor oral hygiene;
  - haematological cancers;
  - liver disease;
  - clotting disorders.

## Management
- Poor oral hygiene.
  - Pink sponges or gauze dipped in mouthwash or water, applied to gums and teeth.

- Clean a furred tongue with a soft toothbrush or with effervescent mouthwash tablets (vitamin C).
  - Use pineapple chunks sucked as sweets to clean the mouth (contains an enzyme ananase).
  - Antiseptic mouth washes or gel, e.g. chlorhexidine.
  - Refer to dentist or hygienist for removal of hard plaque deposits and oral hygiene instruction.
- Oral candidiasis.[1]
  - Nystatin works as a topical agent but not always successful in children due to difficulty getting them to retain solution in mouth.
  - Miconazole gel retains well in the mouth; has both local and systemic effects.
  - Fluconazole: once daily oral agent with high success rate.
- Dry mouth.[2]
  - Correct dehydration.
  - Use humidifier with oxygen.
  - Reassess all medication and rationalize.
  - Apply petroleum jelly, e.g. Vaseline or K-Y jelly, to lips.
  - Stimulate salivation with ice chips, chewing gum, or citrous sweets and drinks.
  - Use artifical saliva such as Glandosanev®.
  - Parasympathomimetics have been used in adult palliative care but there is no experience in children.
- Mouth ulcers:
  - assessment by dentist;
  - antiseptic mouth washes: chlorhexidine;
  - corticosteroids for aphthous ulcers: triamcinolone or hydrocortisone lozenges.
- Bleeding gums.
  - Improve oral hygiene.
  - Tranexamic acid mouth washes.
  - Haemostatic agents: Gelfoam® or Gelfilm®.
  - Platelet transfusion may be required in some haematological disorders/malignancies.

# Feeding

## General points

- Feeding one's child is a basic parental instinct, so a situation where this is causing problems is very distressing not only for the child but also the family.
- Loss of appetite and weight loss occur in many advanced cancers.
- Children with neurological problems experience a lot of difficulties with feeding, including: prolonged feeding time, choking, vomiting, constipation, recurrent chest infections, and poor weight gain.[3]
- Artificial feeding carries many benefits but may also be a burden.
- Artificial feeding is not always perceived by parents as a positive experience.
- The general principles behind the ethics of feeding are discussed in Chapter 3.
- Management of feeding problems should begin with a diagnosis.
- Management of feeding requires a multidisciplinary approach with the major lead coming from dietitians.[4]

## Nutritional assessment

- Assessment of the clinical condition, its state of progression, and the effect of all the different stages on feeding and nutrition.
- Feeding history.
- Social assessment.
- Ability to chew, swallow, and digest.
- Medication review, looking for drugs that affect appetite or taste and drugs that alter absorption of nutrients.
- Serial weight and height measurements.
- Selected laboratory tests.
- Assessment of nutritional requirement of a child should be based on the above and any specific nutritional effects or requirements of their condition.

## Factors that may help when feeding

- Position.
- Seating.
- Feeding equipment.
- Person doing the feeding to be relaxed and calm.
- Positive reinforcement.
- Distraction techniques.
- Accept that feeding may be a lengthy process or time-consuming.
- Alter food:
  - use smaller portions;
  - use smaller plates;
  - encourage more frequent meals;
  - allow parents to give their children 'fast foods';
  - be flexible with timings of meals;
  - make food less effort to eat—mash, soups, etc.
- Involve dietitian early.

- If child experiences abnormal taste:
  - metallic tastes from chemotherapy can be reduced by tart foods such as lemon juice, pickles, etc.;
  - foods with their own flavours such as fruit and boiled sweets;
  - reduce the urea content of diet with specific food.
- Add calorie-rich food to meals, e.g. cheese, cream, etc.
- Energy and nutritional supplements.
- Treat reflux, dyspepsia, constipation, etc.

# Enteral feeding

## Factors that would influence the need for enteral feeding[5]

- Significant risk of aspiration.
- Poor weight gain or weight loss.
- Weight below the 2nd percentile.
- Child unable to swallow food or medication.
- More than 4 hours a day spent on feeding.
- Significant risk of dehydration due to poor swallowing.
- Where the benefits of enteral feeding outweigh the burdens.
- Modifications to feeding regimens can provide solution to some symptoms, such as reflux vomiting. This should ideally always be in collaboration with a dietitian.

## Nasogastric tube

### Benefits
- Cheap.
- Easy to insert: can be done by parents after suitable training.
- Fine bore tube now available.
- Polyurethane tubes can be left in 4–6 weeks before needing changing.
- Does not require hospital admission or general anaesthetic.

### Problems
- Body image.
- Can be traumatic to insert.
- Misplacement in lungs or small intestine.
- Nasal/skin irritation.
- Can be pulled out easily by young children.
- Accidental removal.
- Easily occluded.
- Only medications in a suitable form can be passed down tube.

## Gastrostomy

### Benefits
- Ideal choice for children requiring feeding for more than 3 months.
- Socially more acceptable.
- Less likely to be taken out or fall out.
- Can be used for overnight feeding.
- Management is easy for parents.
- Experience of fitting now developed by many paediatric surgeons with excellent results.

### Problems
- Occlusion.
- Granulation tissue formation.
- Requires general anaesthetic to fit (new technique of using radiologically inserted gastrostomy without general anaesthetic in adults has now started being used in teenagers).
- Infection.
- Tube can fall or be pulled out.
- Body image.

- If gastro-oesophageal reflux present then may require fundoplication.[6]
- Only medications in a suitable form can be passed down tube.

## Gastrostomy blockage[7]

In the event of a blockage the following can be tried. Using a 50mL syringe (smaller syringes can create too great a pressure and damage the tube) the following fluids (25–30mL) can be used (as age-appropriate) to unblock the tube, usually a minimum of 10mL.

- Flush with warm water.
- Flush with soda water.
- Flush with cola or pineapple juice.
- Try gently drawing back on syringe.
- Squeeze along the length (milking) of the tube.
- For a PEG, use pancreatic enzyme (Pancrex V®), instil, and leave for 30min.
- For Mic-Key, consider changing the tube.

# Hydration

## General points

- Hydration in the palliative care setting is normally via oral or enteral route.
- Children in the terminal phase of their illness can often be left mildly fluid-restricted to reduce terminal secretion.
- The younger the child, the less well they tolerate variations of fluid balance.
- Fluid balance is based on weight and not age.
- The calculation in the box is based on APLS recommendations.[8]

## References

**1** Lavy, V. (2007). Presenting symptoms and signs in children referred for palliative care in Malawi. *Palliative Med.* **21** (4), 333–9.

**2** Duval, M. and Wood, C. (2002). [Treatment of non-painful symptoms in terminally ill children]. *Arch. Pediatr.* **9** (11), 1173–8.

**3** Sullivan, P.B., Lambert, B., Rose, M., Ford-Adams, M., Griffiths, P., and Johnson, A. (2000). Prevalence and severity of feeding and nutritional problems in children with neurological impairment: Oxford Feeding Study. *Dev. Med. Child Neurol.* **42** (10), 674–80.

**4** Ayoob, K.T. and Barresi, I. (2007). Feeding disorders in children: taking an interdisciplinary approach. *Pediatr. Ann.* **36** (8), 478–83.

**5** Motion, S., Northstone, K., Emond, A., Stucke, S., and Golding, J. (2002). Early feeding problems in children with cerebral palsy: weight and neurodevelopmental outcomes. *Dev. Med. Child Neurol.* **44** (1), 40–3.

**6** Samuel, M. and Holmes, K. (2002). Quantitative and qualitative analysis of gastroesophageal reflux after percutaneous endoscopic gastrostomy. *J. Pediatr. Surg.* **37** (2), 256–61.

**7** Jassal, S, (2007). *Basic symptom control in paediatric palliative care, the Rainbows Children's Hospice guidelines*, 7th edn. Rainbows Children's Hospice, Loughborough.

**8** Advanced Life Support Group (2005). *Advanced paediatric life support*, 4th edn. BMJ Books, London.

# Dyspnoea

# Introduction

The principles that underlie management of dyspnoea are the same as those underlying management of any other symptom namely:
- holistic;
- rational;
- balancing burden and benefit.

## Holistic approach

Dyspnoea is defined as the sense that breathing has become unpleasant. It is therefore by definition a subjective phenomenon. It also means that many different factors can contribute to dyspnoea. These include:
- physical factors (fluid, tumour, weakness, injury);
- psychosocial factors (fears about function, inability to carry out normal tasks such as walking or feeding);
- existential or spiritual (interference with respiratory function carries implication of imminent death, fear of suffocation).

### Dyspnoea is subjective

It is important to remember that there is only limited correlation between the observation of disordered breathing (e.g. tachypnoea) and the experience of dyspnoea. Breathing can be unpleasant without being abnormal, and can be abnormal without being unpleasant.

The multidimensional significance of difficulty in breathing is highlighted by the dual meanings of the terms 'inspire' and 'expire'. The word 'spirit' itself is related both to breath and to the essence of life. The sensation that breathing has ceased to be effortless and has become unpleasant or difficult carries with it emotional weight that goes well beyond the physical. Conversely, breathing that is abnormal to the observer may not be unpleasant. An obvious example is the tachypnoea associated with ketoacidosis.

# Pathophysiology

It is helpful to consider the possible causes for dyspnoea by considering in turn all the parts of the respiratory system from diaphragm to respiratory centre.

### Muscle weakness
- Causes:
  - cachexia;
  - Duchenne muscular dystrophy;
  - other neuromuscular degenerative conditions.
- Interventions:
  - not always possible to intervene effectively;
  - nocturnal ventilation;
  - management of cachexia.

### Fluid in respiratory tree
- Causes:
  - secretions;
  - infection.
- Interventions:
  - antibiotics;
  - anticholinergics;

▶ Effects of antiobiotics and anticholinergics are mutually counterproductive. Anticholinergics reduce volume of secretions, but increase their viscosity, which may interfere with mucociliary clearance. Antibiotics may improve infection but carry their own adverse effects. The best approach needs individual assessment, taking into account priorities of child and family.

### Pressure on airway
- Cause: tumour.
- Interventions:
  - steroids;
  - radiotherapy;
  - palliative chemotherapy;
  - stent.
- Parenchymal metastatic lung disease is rarely symptomatic and does not usually need intervention.
- Management should be in close collaboration with paediatric oncology and radiotherapy colleagues.
- Long-term steroid therapy should usually be avoided.
- Surgical insertion of stent is invasive and often not appropriate.

### Pain
- Causes:
  - metastatic bone disease in ribs;
  - inflammation (e.g. pleuritic reaction);
  - rubbing of ribs on pelvis in extreme kyphoscoliosis.

- Interventions: good analgesic management using opioids and appropriate adjuvants such as NSAIDs, bisphosphonates, radiotherapy, etc.

## Pneumothorax or effusion
- Cause: usually malignant.
- Interventions:
  - analgesia;
  - pleural drainage;
  - pleuradesis.
- Pleural drainage in children usually demands admission to hospital and specialist anaesthetic and surgical involvement.
- Malignant effusions usually reaccumulate within a few days or at most weeks.
- Pleuradesis is painful in a significant minority of cases.
- Pleuradesis is unsuccessful in a significant minority of cases.

## Cough and haemoptysis
- Causes:
  - infection;
  - tumour;
- Interventions for cough:
  - inhaled local anaesthetic agents have been used in adults, but are poorly tolerated in children and risk aspiration through impairment of gag reflex;
  - opioids;
  - radiotherapy (see 'Interventions for haemoptysis' below).
- Interventions for haemoptysis:
  - haemoptysis frightening for child and family; should usually treat;
  - reassurance that major haemorrhage is, in reality, unlikely;
  - radiotherapy has dual effect of shrinking tumour and reducing bleeding from surface;
  - haemoptysis usually caused by tumour pressing on major airway; parenchymal tumour or metastasis is rarely the cause;
  - etamsylate and tranexamic acid can both reduce the risk of haemoptysis;
  - prepare for possibility of larger haemorrhage, including parenteral midazolam; ensure dark green surgical towels are by child's bedside.

## Upper airway secretions ('death rattle')
- Occurs in last 24–48 hours of life.
- Usually occurs in comatose patient who is unaware.
- Symptom is distressing for friends and family at the child's bedside and therefore should be treated.
- Interventions:
  - reduce any parenteral fluids to 50% maintenance; reassure family that this will not in any way shorten child's life;
  - anticholinergics (e.g. hyoscine patch or via subcutaneous syringe driver) reduce the volume but increase the viscosity of secretions;
  - suction can be uncomfortable in child who is still aware, but can be valued by the family as an intervention they can carry out.

# Other causes of dyspnoea

## Claustrophobia

- Causes:
  - inability to take a deep breath (e.g. due to muscle weakness);
  - presence of oxygen mask on the face;
  - use of BiPAP or NIPPV.
- Interventions:
  - movement of air on the face (e.g. open window, switch on electric fan);
  - consider need for or appropriateness of face mask.

## Hypoxia

- Many and various causes, particularly in the final hours of life.
- Hypoxia should only be treated if symptomatic. Oxygen saturation monitors in the final days and weeks of life offer little benefit for most families.
- Oxygen does not relieve dyspnoea in the absence of hypoxaemia.[1]
- The need for oxygen in the palliative phase should be considered very carefully for the individual child and family.

## Fear

The fear associated with difficulty in breathing leads to a powerful vicious cycle in which difficulty breathing reinforces anxiety, which in turn exacerbates difficulty in breathing. An ascending spiral of anxiety may result in a 'panic attack'.

### Interventions

- Adequate exploration of fears and, where appropriate, reassurance.
- Elementary breathing techniques aimed at putting child and family back in control of the breathing.
- Complementary therapies (e.g. hypnosis).
- Opioids. There are opioid receptors in the respiratory and cough centres of the brain. Doses of opioid effective for dyspnoea are approximately 50% of those required for pain. Otherwise, principles of prescription and titration are precisely the same.
- Benzodiazepines. Benzodiazepines act on receptors in higher centres to relieve anxiety, and on receptors in the respiratory centre. Long acting benzodiazepines such as lorazepam and diazepam can be useful for background dyspnoea. Buccal or parenteral midazolam is particularly useful for intervening in acute episodes of dyspnoea or panic attacks.
- Nebulized saline. Some patients derive benefit from nebulized saline. The mechanism is not clear, but may be a combination of dilution of viscid secretions and the effect of blowing on the face.
- Reversible causes. An element of reversible bronchoconstriction is not uncommon even in terminal dyspnoea and may be improved by $B_2$ agonists. Symptomatic pulmonary congestion due to cardiac failure may improve with diuretics.

- Other nebulized medications. The evidence for benefit of nebulized opioids in adults or in children is slight.[2] However, they do little or no harm and individual patients sometimes report benefit. It is unclear whether this benefit is separable from that of blowing on the face. Nebulized mucolytics provide symptom benefit in cystic fibrosis.

# Management

## Steps in managing dyspnoea

1  Consider the possibility of dyspnoea and proactively ask about it.
2  Where practical, establish in discussion with the child whether breathing problems are a concern to him or herself.
3  Explore what the breathing difficulties 'mean' to the child and family.
4  Take a careful history of the nature of the symptom.
5  Perform a careful examination.
6  Make a rational diagnosis of the cause(s) for dyspnoea.
7  Construct a rational therapeutic approach, weighing each intervention carefully with respect to potential good it may do and the potential harm.
8  Review the effectiveness of the intervention.

## Decision-making

Because dyspnoea is a subjective symptom that correlates only poorly with observed abnormal parameters, it is critical to engage the child and family in a discussion before embarking on a therapeutic strategy. All interventions carry the risk of adverse as well as beneficial effects, and it is not justifiable to commence an intervention to solve a problem that exists only in the eye of the observer.

A special example of this is the use of noninvasive positive-pressure ventilation (NIPPV). There is now good evidence that this can improve symptoms and quality of life in many life-limited children.[3,4] Nevertheless, for some individual children and young people, the NIPPV itself is an intolerable burden.

Like all palliative manoeuvres, NIPPV and other interventions for dyspnoea should be carried out only when the benefit to the patient (and sometimes the family) outweighs the burden.

## References

**1** Uronis, H.E., Currow, D.C., McCrory, D.C., Samsa, G.P., and Abernethy, A.P. (2008). Oxygen for relief of dyspnoea in mildly- or non-hypoxaemic patients with cancer: a systematic review and meta-analysis. *Br. J. Cancer* **98** (2), 294–9.

**2** Currow, D.C. and Abernethy, A.P. (2007). Pharmacological management of dyspnoea. *Curr. Opin. Support. Palliative Care* **1** (2), 96–101.

**3** Mellies, U., Dohna-Schwake, C., Stehling, F., and Voit, T. (2004). Sleep disordered breathing in spinal muscular atrophy. *Neuromuscul. Disord.* **14** (12), 797–803.

**4** Young, A.C., Wilson, J.W., Kotsimbos, T.C., and Naughton, M.T. (2008). Randomised placebo controlled trial of non-invasive ventilation for hypercapnia in cystic fibrosis. *Thorax* **63** (1), 72–7.

# Neurological symptoms

# Epilepsy

**Definition** Recurrent convulsive or non-convulsive seizures caused by partial or generalized epileptogenic discharges in the cerebrum.

## General points

- Not all seizures are grand-mal epileptic seizures; they come in many forms and it is important to recognize the different types.
- Not all seizures require immediate administration of medication. The majority of seizures will settle given 5–10min, particularly in children with neurodegenerative disorders.
- Look for the reversible causes of increased seizures and attempt to correct them.
- Seizures can be very frightening for the child, family, and carers. Try to remain calm, give parents an explanation of what is happening, and treat the child in a logical manner.

## Reversible causes of increased seizures

- Infection.
- Renal failure.
- Hepatic failure.
- Electrolyte imbalance (sodium, calcium, or magnesium).
- Hypoglycaemia.
- Raised intracranial pressure.
- Inappropriate epilepsy management.
- Too rapid an increase or decrease of epilepsy medication.

## General principles of management[1,2]

- Correctly diagnose the type of epileptic seizure.[2,3]
- Know which drugs are used to treat the different types of seizures (Table 13.1).
- Start with one drug, working up the dose gradually until seizure control or side effects occur.[2]
- Add second drug only if seizure control not achieved with first drug alone.
- Remember to weigh up the benefits versus side effects of the treatments. 30% of children have behavioural problems whilst on anticonvulsants.[5,6]
- Change doses gradually.
- Regular recalculation of drug dosage as the child grows and puts on weight.
- Metabolism of drugs can be affected by hepatic and renal failure.[7]
- Children under the age of 3 years may need higher doses of drugs due to their more efficient drug metabolism.
- Blood levels are generally unhelpful.
- If in doubt ask a paediatric neurologist.

**Table 13.1** Antiepileptic drugs*

| Drugs | Advantages | Disadvantages | Comments |
|---|---|---|---|
| Carbamazepine | Effective for partial and tonic-clonic seizures, minimal side effects | Transient adverse effects during initiation; no parenteral formulation; may worsen absence seizures; complex pharmacokinetics. Drowsiness, coordination problems, & extrapyramidal movements | Drug of 1st choice for partial epilepsies |
| Ethosuximide | Effective for absence seizures; few side effects | Only for absence seizures; frequent GI symptoms | 1st choice drug for absence seizures |
| Phenobarbital | Broad spectrum of efficacy | Sedative, cognitive, or behavioural effects; hyperkinetic behaviour | Not 1st choice drug but safe & cheap; useful in cerebral irritation |
| Phenytoin | Effective: partial & tonic-colonic seizures; parenteral formulation | Cosmetic or dysmorphic side effects; saturation kinetics | Another 1st choice drug for partial epilepsies; potent enzyme inhibitor |
| Primidone | Effective: partial & tonic-colonic seizures | Toxicity; behavioural effects, drowsiness, ataxia, personality changes | Not 1st choice drug |
| Valproate (valproic acid) | Broad spectrum of efficacy | Weight gain, tremor, ataxia, drowsiness | 1st choice drug for idiopathic epilepsy; an alternative for partial seizures |
| Gabapentin | Effective in partial & tonic-colonic seizures, well tolerated | Limited absorption, short half-life, moderate efficacy. Somnolence | Mechanism of action unknown; additional use as adjuvant in neuropathic pain |

**Table 13.1** (*Contd.*)

| Lamotrigine | Broad spectrum, sense of well being | Hypersensitivity reaction rash, metabolism inducible; dizziness, ataxia, somnolence | |
| --- | --- | --- | --- |
| Vigabatrin | Effective: partial & tonic-colonic seizures, infantile spasms | Eye problems, dyskinesias | Unique mechanism of action |

* Data from Mattson, R.H. (1996). The role of the old and the new antiepileptic drugs in special populations: mental and multiple handicaps. *Epilepsia* **37** (Suppl. 6), S45–53.

# Intractable epilepsy

The management of intractable epilepsy is beyond the scope of this manual. However it is worth remembering a few points.[2,8–12]

- 40% of children with intractable epilepsy are misdiagnosed. This can be due to:-
  - underlying aetiology overlooked;
  - misdiagnosis of syndrome or seizure type;
  - poor EEG recording or interpretation;
  - non-epileptic disorders that mimic epileptic disorders.
- There are often errors in therapy due to:-
  - inappropriate choice of drugs;
  - inappropriate dose and dosing interval;
  - inappropriate polytherapy.
- *In all cases of intractable epilepsy check*:-
  - that child has actually seen a paediatric neurologist and has had a formal diagnosis of type of epilepsy;
  - if on polytherapy, has this decision been made by a paediatric neurologist and, if not, what is the rationale for the polytherapy?

# Status epilepticus

**Definition** When seizures occur so frequently that, over the course of 30 or more minutes, patients have not recovered from the coma produced by one attack, before the next attack supervenes.

**Management**[13]

In the community or smaller units (major hospitals have established protocols that should be followed):
- secure airway;
- give oxygen;
- establish cause;
- check for hypoglycaemia;
- if facilities available, check FBC, U & E, glucose, calcium, magnesium, liver function tests, blood cultures. If possible check urine for infection.

*First line treatment*[14–16]

*Diazepam*
- iv: getting new access site is difficult, onset of action in 1–3min, effective in 80% of cases within 5min, short duration of action 15–20min.
- pr: as a solution (suppositories take too long to work) works within 6–8min.
- NG tube or gastrostomy: best mode if available.

*Midazolam*
- Buccally: increasingly popular due to ease of administration, works within 6–8min.
- pr.

*Lorazepam*
- iv: as infusion; give slowly to avoid apnoea.
- pr.
- po.
- Sublingually.

The metabolites of diazepam are active. Furthermore, diazepam accumulates in lipid stores. When these stores saturate, then the levels rise rapidly leading to unexpected side effects (secondary peak phenomenon). This is not true of lorazepam.

**Second line treatment** If still fitting then repeat first line treatment after 10–15min.

**Third line treatment**
If there is still no response then rectal paraldehyde should be administered.

Paraldehyde should be mixed in an equal volume of arachis oil (or olive oil if there is any nut allergy), drawn up into a glass syringe, and given via a quill (if urgent, a plastic syringe can be used provided it is drawn up and given immediately).

**Fourth line treatment**
Hospitalize the child for advanced management, paralysis, and ventilation.

# Terminal seizures or if not appropriate to hospitalize

In the terminal phase seizures can become more severe and frequent. The child at this stage is normally not able to take or absorb oral anti-epileptics, and in such cases continuous sc midazolam or phenobarbital can be used. The physician needs to balance the heavily sedating effects of treatment against the benefits of seizure control. It may not be possible to control all the seizures, and it is necessary to explain to the parents that some minor seizures may break through and do not necessarily require escalation of treatment.

## Midazolam sc infusion[14–16]

- Onset of action 1–5min.
- Duration of action 1–5h.
- Easier to titrate than phenobarbital.
- Good anxiolytic.
- Dose can be steadily increased (up to 150mg/24h then consider changing to phenobarbital).
- Only available in one strength so volume in smaller Graseby syringe drivers can be a problem.
- Anecdotal evidence suggests that a small dose of diamorphine added to syringe driver can help with seizures requiring increasing doses of midazolam.
- Clonazepam is an alternate to midazolam.

## Phenobarbital sc infusion

- Sedating.
- Anxiolytic.
- Do not combine with other drugs in syringe driver (only miscible with diamorphine and hyoscine).
- Should be diluted with water.

# Spasticity

**Definition** A condition of increased tone, spasms, clonus, weakness, and loss of dexterity.

## Causes
- Cerebral palsy.
- Brain haemorrhage.
- Brain tumours.
- Anoxia.
- Vegetative state.

## Management[17]
- Multidisciplinary.
- Physiotherapy.
- Surgical.
- Botulinum A injections.[18]
- Drugs:[19] not always very successful:
  - baclofen, orally or by pump;
  - diazepam;
  - tizanidine;
  - dantrolene;
  - quinine;
  - gabapentin.

# Myoclonus

**Definition** Brief, abrupt, involuntary, non-suppressible, and jerky contractions involving a single muscle or muscle group.[20]

## Causes
- Normal; onset of sleep, exercise, anxiety.
- Neurodegenerative disorders.
- Secondary to opioid overdose.

## Management
- Opioid rotation (see Chapter 7).
- Benzodiazepines:
  - diazepam;
  - lorazepam;
  - clonazepam.

# Chorea

**Definition** Frequent, brief, purposeless movements that tend to flow from body part to body part chaotically and unpredictably.[20]

## Causes
- Rheumatic fever.
- Neurodegenerative disorder.
- Encephalopathy.
- Hypo- and hypernatraemia.
- Drugs including:[21]
  - haloperidol;
  - phenytoin;
  - phenothiazines.

## Management
- Bed rest in quiet darkened room.
- Sodium valproate.

# Dystonia

**Definition** Syndrome of sustained muscle contractions, frequently causing twisting and repetitive movements or abnormal postures.[20]

## Causes
- Neurodegenerative disorders.
- Metabolic disorders.
- In drug-induced reactions producing extrapyramidal reactions.
- Drugs including:[21]
  - dopamine antagonists;
  - antipsychotics;
  - antiemetics;
  - antidepressants;
  - antiepileptics.

## Management
- Anticholinergic drugs such as benztropine or diphenhydramine (in collaboration with neurologist).
- Review medication and reduce or stop drugs if possible.

# Akathisia

**Definition** Motor restlessness, in which the patient feels compelled to pace up and down, or to change body position frequently.[20]

**Causes** Drugs including haloperidol and prochlorperazine.[21]

**Management**
- Review medication and reduce or stop drugs if possible.
- Propranolol.

## References

**1** Shinnar, S. and Pellock, J.M. (2002). Update on the epidemiology and prognosis of pediatric epilepsy. *J. Child Neurol.* **17** (Suppl. 1), S4–17.

**2** Udani, V. (2000). Evaluation and management of intractable epilepsy. *Indian J. Pediatr.* **67** (1 Suppl.), S61–70.

**3** Murphy, J.V. and Dehkharghani, F. (1994). Diagnosis of childhood seizure disorders. *Epilepsia* **35** (Suppl. 2:), S7–17.

**4** Mattson, R.H. (1996). The role of the old and the new antiepileptic drugs in special populations: mental and multiple handicaps. *Epilepsia* **37** (Suppl. 6), S45–53.

**5** Dunn, D.W. (2003). Neuropsychiatric aspects of epilepsy in children. *Epilepsy Behav.* **4** (2), 101–6.

**6** Holmes, G.L., Chevassus-Au-Lois, N., Sarkisian, M.R., and Ben-Ari, Y. (1997). [Consequences of recurrent seizures during development]. *Rev. Neurol.* **25** (141), 749–53.

**7** Anderson, G.D. (2002). Children versus adults: pharmacokinetic and adverse-effect differences. *Epilepsia* **43** (Suppl. 3), 53–9.

**8** Blume, W.T. (1992). Uncontrolled epilepsy in children. *Epilepsy Res. Suppl.* **5**, 19–24.

**9** Camfield, P.R. and Camfield, C.S. (1996). Antiepileptic drug therapy: when is epilepsy truly intractable? *Epilepsia* **37** (Suppl. 1), S60–5.

**10** Holmes, G.L. (1993). Seizure disorders in children. *Curr. Opin. Pediatr.* **5** (6), 653–9.

**11** Iinuma, K. (1999). [General principles of treatment and effects of childhood intractable epilepsy]. *Rinsho Shinkeigaku* **39** (1), 75–6.

**12** Steinborn, B. (2000). [Intractable epilepsy of childhood and its treatment]. *Neurol. Neurochir. Pol.* **33** (Suppl. 1), 37–48.

**13** Mitchell, W.G. (1996). Status epilepticus and acute repetitive seizures in children, adolescents, and young adults: etiology, outcome, and treatment. *Epilepsia* **37** (Suppl. 1), S74–80.

**14** Camfield, P.R. (1999). Buccal midazolam and rectal diazepam for treatment of prolonged seizures in childhood and adolescence: a randomised trial. *J. Pediatr.* **135** (3), 398–9.

**15** Grimshaw, D., Holyroyd, E., Anthony, D., and Hall, D.M. (1995). Subcutaneous midazolam, diamorphine and hyoscine infusion in palliative care of a child with neurodegenerative disease. *Child Care Health Dev.* **21** (6), 377–81.

**16** Scott, R.C., Besag, F.M., and Neville, B.G. (1999). Buccal midazolam and rectal diazepam for treatment of prolonged seizures in childhood and adolescence: a randomised trial. *Lancet* **353** (9153), 623–6.

**17** Gormley, M.E., Jr., Krach, L.E., and Piccini, L. (2001). Spasticity management in the child with spastic quadriplegia. *Eur. J. Neurol.* **8** (Suppl. 5), 127–35.

**18** Koman, L.A., Paterson Smith, B., and Balkrishnan, R. (2003). Spasticity associated with cerebral palsy in children: guidelines for the use of botulinum A toxin. *Paediatr. Drugs* **5** (1), 11–23.

**19** Krach, L.E. (2001). Pharmacotherapy of spasticity: oral medications and intrathecal baclofen. *J. Child Neurol.* **16** (1), 31–6.

**20** Schlaggar, B.L. and Mink, J.W. (2003). Movement disorders in children. *Pediatr. Rev.* **24** (2), 39–51.

**21** Twycross, R. (2002). In *Palliative care formulary* (ed. A.W.R. Twycross, S. Charlesworth, and A. Dickman), p. 339. Radcliffe Medical Press, Oxford.

# Psychological symptoms

# Introduction

Disorders of the psyche (particularly depression and anxiety) are relatively common among children with life-limiting conditions. Most of the tools available for evaluating or assessing them in palliative medicine were developed for adults, as were strategies for treating them.[1]

Although ideal practice would be to collaborate with local child and adolescent mental health services in the management of all such children,[2] service provision in most areas is such that this is rarely practical in children's palliative care. Nevertheless, where there is ready access to such services, advice should be sought.

# Depression: general points

- Despite the extensive literature on child psychiatry and psychology there is very little on psychological symptoms in paediatric palliative care.
- The standard DSM-IV and ICD-10 scales for assessing depression are inappropriate for assessing depression in paediatric palliative care.
- Most other tools for diagnosing depression do not take into account illness in the child.
- The clinical picture is dependent on the condition and developmental age of the child.
- There may be reluctance in clinicians diagnosing psychological problems[3] due to:
  - concern over adding an additional burden of another condition on to the child and family;
  - belief that that reaction is normal under the circumstances of their existing condition;
  - concerns around the doctor's own ability to diagnose and manage psychological problems;
  - belief that only an expert psychiatrist, psychologist, or counsellor can recognize this type of problem.
- Children can have adjustment reactions (regression, enuresis, etc.) to serious illness and it can be difficult to differentiate this from depression. However adjustment reaction normally occurs within 3 months of the stressor and does not last longer than 6 months.
- The risk of developing psychological problems is also linked to :
  - pre-existing psychosocial factors;
  - maternal psychiatric/psychological state.
- Children with a life-limiting condition appear to report less depression than expected. This may be due to repression.
  - Repression is a form of denial used by children (often adolescents) as a form of coping mechanism when dealing with their illness. This is often seen as a continually changing pattern of acceptance and denial.
  - Repression appears to be a long-term behaviour pattern.

# Managing depression

## General principles
- The best tools in terms of diagnosis are:
  - listening to the child, family, and multidisciplinary team with care and compassion;
  - time, both in terms of the assessment, but also being prepared to talk when the child feels ready to open up; good care will require regular meetings with the child and family;
  - structured clinical interview;
  - understanding of the natural progression of the life-limiting condition and the effects this can have on the child (e.g. muscular dystrophy child who develops loss of mobility and independence at the same time as developing awareness of illness/death and entering adolescence).
- For psychological problems it is not necessary for a doctor or specialist counsellor to tackle all the issues. The child may not choose to open up to the doctor but may well disclose their feelings to nurses, teachers, or religious leaders. It is important to support all these groups.
- Understand the stresses and strains in the family.
- Appreciate that the child may feel frightened and guilty about their illness and how it affects their family.
- Give honest answers to straight questions.
- Open communication and allowing the child to be involved in their management is very helpful.
- Medication only forms one part of the support that the child and family may need.
- Treatment should involve psychological therapies, including counselling and complementary therapies.
- Cognitive behavioural therapy has been shown to be very effective in the normal paediatric population but its benefit in life-limited children is mainly anecdotal.
- Depression and anxiety are often interlinked, so assessment must encompass both.
- Be prepared to seek advice from a child psychiatrist.

## Pharmacological approach
- There are essentially two groups of drugs that are used to treat depression: tricyclic antidepressants and selective serotonin re-uptake inhibitors (SSRI).
- ▶ The safety and efficacy of drugs used in the treatment of depression in children has not been established; long-term safety information is also lacking.[4]
- The use of antidepressants is determined by the individual child's medical condition, medications, psychiatric state, and risk of suicide.
- Initiation of treatment should be made after open and honest discussion with the child, family, and care team. Very few children or parents will say no to medication if it is truly required.

- Hyponatraemia has been associated with antidepressants (particularly SSRI). This should be considered in any child who develops unexpected drowsiness, confusion, or convulsions whilst on antidepressants.
- Rapid withdrawal of antidepressants can cause nausea, vomiting, anorexia, headaches, and giddiness. Any child on medication for over 8 weeks should have this withdrawn slowly.

*Tricyclic antidepressants*
- Dosages for antidepressant benefit have to be sufficiently high; however at that level side effects often limit their benefit.
- These can be split into two groups: sedating (amitriptyline) and non-sedating (imipramine).
- The main concerns centre around antimuscarinic and cardiac side effects.
- Side effects include:
  - arrythmias;
  - heart block;
  - convulsions—use with caution in epilepsy;
  - drowsiness;
  - dry mouth;
  - blurred vision;
  - constipation;
  - urinary retention;
  - suicidal thoughts/behaviour.

*Selective serotonin re-uptake inhibitors*
- The CSM has advised that the risk and benefit balance for the following SSRIs is considered unfavourable in the under 18 year olds: citalopram, escitalopram, paroxetine, and sertraline.[5,6]
- Only fluoxetine has shown to be effective in treating depression in children.[7]
- The risk from SSRIs appears to be related to suicidal thoughts and behaviour (there have been no confirmed deaths). This risk is particularly high in the first few weeks of treatment.
- SSRIs can cause an increase in anxiety in the first 2–4 weeks of treatment.
- It can take up to 4 weeks to see an improvement in a child and up to 6–8 weeks to see maximum benefit from medication.
- Use with caution in children with epilepsy, cardiac disease, diabetes mellitus, history of mania, or bleeding disorders.
- Side effects are similar to those of tricyclics but there tend to be less sedating and fewer antimuscarinic effects, although nausea and anxiety is greater in the first few weeks.

# Anxiety

## General points

- Anxiety can come from a number of different sources:[8]
  - separation anxiety;
  - procedure-related;
  - death anxiety;
  - inpatient admission (abandonment);
  - receiving bad news.
- As with depression, doctors may be reluctant to diagnose, as they see the behaviour as normal under the circumstances.
- Diagnostic tools tend to be unhelpful.
- Maternal psychiatric disorder increases the risk of anxiety in the child.
- Over the development age of 10 years almost all children are aware of their prognosis, whether they have been told by parents/doctors or not.[9]
- Anxiety is significantly reduced if the child is openly told, in terms they understand, about their condition.
- Death anxiety is greatest in children whose development age is between 6 and 10 years.

## General principles of management

See Chapter 14, Managing depression, p. 156.

- Good communication skills and allowing the child to express their anxiety are important.
- Music therapy, art therapy, massage, reflexology, hypnosis, and acupuncture have all been shown to be very effective in managing a range of different types of anxiety.
- Cognitive behavioural therapy has been shown to be effective in the normal paediatric population but its benefits in paediatric palliative care have only been proved in procedural pain.
- Look at the developmental age of the child when assessing symptoms.
- Remember to treat the family as well as the child.
- Prevention is better than cure; pre-plan before procedures.

## Pharmacological approach

- Benzodiazepines are the main group of drugs used to treat short-term anxiety.[10]
- The type of benzodiazepine used is dependent on the nature and type of anxiety symptom.
- They are best used as short-term treatments.
- For more chronic anxiety states, antidepressant medication should be used.
- Benzodiazepines are particularly helpful in the first few weeks when SSRIs are started.

### Benzodiazepines

*Midazolam*

- Fast acting.
- Can be given by the intranasal, subcutaneous, oral, or buccal route.

- Intranasal can cause nasal irritation.
- Now comes in a flavoured buccal preparation.
- Is particularly useful in the anxious dying child or for procedural anxiety.
- Can rarely cause paradoxical agitation.

*Lorazepam*
- Fast acting.
- Can be given by the sublingual, oral, or rectal route.
- The injection solution can be used for the sublingual or rectal route.
- The tablet is particularly useful in the older child as it is easy to carry around and can be used orally or sublingually.
- Is particularly useful in the anxious dying child or for procedural anxiety.

*Diazepam*
- Slow acting when taken orally.
- Longer acting than midazolam or lorazepam.
- Can develop cumulative effect where repeated dosages can cause sudden heavy sedation.

### Tricyclic antidepressants and SSRIs
- See Chapter 14, Managing depression, p. 156.
- Fluoxetine is the drug of choice for generalized anxiety.[11]

# Insomnia

Insomnia is a problem not only for the child but also the parents.

## Causes

It is important to address the possible causes for insomnia before embarking on medication:

- fear and/or anxiety;
- underlying depression;
- disturbed night-time routine from giving medication or conducting procedures;
- pain, discomfort, or side effects of medication or feeding;
- altered biorhythms with the child sleeping during the day due to medication causing sedation or child's/family's routine (e.g. parents putting child to sleep during the day so they can have a break);
- the disease process itself; many neurodegenerative conditions are linked to altered or diminished sleep patterns.

## General principles of management

- Identify anxiety or depression and manage appropriately.
- Look at the sleep pattern and try to devise a routine before bed time to help relax the child down, such as warm bath, story, darkened room, etc.
- Alter drug timing to reduce night disturbances as much as possible.
- Change any medication that may cause problems in the night (e.g. NSAIDs and dyspepsia at night).
- Consider complementary therapies such as aromatherapy or massage for both the child and also the parents.
- Develop a realistic expectation of how long the child can or needs to sleep with the parents.
- Accept that adolescents may choose to go to sleep very late at night and sleep in.

## Pharmacological approach

The use of medication should be considered as a last resort for insomnia when all other approaches have failed. A number of different drugs can be used for insomnia.

### Chloral derivatives[12]

- Chloral hydrate and triclofos were formerly popular hypnotics in children.
- Triclofos causes fewer gastrointestinal side effects.
- Chloral derivatives are soporific (i.e. promote sleep) but not anxiolytic.

### Temazepam

- A long acting benzodiazepine now used extensively, particularly for the older child.
- Works for 4–6h.
- Should be taken up to 1h before bedtime.

*Promethazine*
- An antihistamine.
- Sedative effects can diminish after a few days of continued use.

*Melatonin*[13,14]
- A pineal hormone that affects sleep patterns.
- Used for sleep disorder in children with cerebral palsy, attention deficit disorder, and autism.
- Increasingly being tried out of licence for children with neurodegenerative conditions.
- Should be initiated and supervised by specialists.

# Terminal delirium

Delirium, often called acute confusion state, can be seen at any stage through a child's illness but is more prevalent at the terminal stage.

## Clinical features

- Terminal restlessness.
- Acute onset.
- Fluctuating nature.
- Disorientation.
- Agitation or lethargy.
- Altered perception.
- Auditory or visual hallucinations.
- Potentially reversible.

## Causes

- Drugs:
  - opioids;
  - antimuscarinics;
  - corticosteroids.
- Drug withdrawal.
- Cerebral disease:
  - hypoxia;
  - sepsis;
  - primary or secondary cancers;
  - cerebral vascular accident.
- Anxiety or depression.
- Pain.
- Constipation.
- Organ failure:
  - liver;
  - kidney.
- Biochemical:
  - hypercalcaemia;
  - hyponatraemia;
  - hyperosmolality.
- Infection:
  - urinary;
  - respiratory;
  - neurological;
  - other causes of septicaemia.
- Nutritional deficiencies.

## General principles of management

- Assess fully; identify reversible causes, and manage appropriately.
- Reassure the family and the child by explaining what is happening.
- Repeat important information to the child.
- Set a calm environment for the child:
  - reduce noise;
  - adequate lighting;
  - have family around child;

- use familiar staff to care for the child;
- use bedding, toys, and comfort items that the child is familiar with.
- Do not use any forms of restraint.

## Pharmacological approach

From the onset it is important to establish what you hope to achieve with medication. The plan should be to help improve the mental state whilst controlling sedation. This is not always achievable.

There is no research available for the use of drugs to manage delirium in paediatric palliative care. Treatments used are extrapolated from adult palliative care.

Two main groups of drugs are used, phenothiazines and benzodiazepines, but phenobarbital also deserves a special mention.

### Phenothiazines

- Haloperidol is the drug of choice in delirium.[15]
  - It is a potent neuroleptic with antidopaminergic activity.
  - It has relative few anti-cholinergic side effects.
  - Extrapyramidal reactions occur rarely at higher doses.
  - It improves cognition.
  - It has sedative effects at higher doses.
  - It can be given by the po, sc, iv, or im route.
  - It is fast acting within hours.
  - It combines with benzodiazepines for rapid sedation.
- Levomepromazine.
  - It is a potent neuroleptic with antidopamine activity.
  - Used as an antiemetic in children.
  - In higher doses it can be used to induce sedation.

### Benzodiazepines

- Midazolam or lorazepam are the drugs of choice.
- They should not be used alone as they may worsen delirium.[16]
- They do not improve cognition but only induce sedation.
- They combine well with haloperidol.
- They can be given by the po, sublingual, buccal, pr, sc, or iv route.
- At higher doses they can cause paradoxical agitation and delirium.
- Children with neurodegenerative disorders are already often on benzodiazepines for their epilepsy and these children can tolerate high doses of benzodiazepines.

### Phenobarbital[17]

- Phenobarbital can be used as second line treatment.
- It can help control symptoms of agitation.
- Particularly good if anticonvulsant action required.
- Elevates seizure threshold (phenothiazines lower threshold).
- If used as sc infusion, it should be used as sole agent with regular assessment of the insertion site as it can cause skin irritation.

## References

1 Kelly, B., McClement, S., and Chochinov, H.M. (2006). Measurement of psychological distress in palliative care. *Palliative Med.* **20** (8), 779–89.

2 NICE (2005). *Depression in children and young people: identification and management in primary, community and secondary care*, clinical guidelines CG28. NICE, London.

3 Froese, A.P. (1977). Pediatric referrals to psychiatry: III. Is the psychiatrist's opinion heard? *Int. J. Psychiatry Med.* **8** (3), 295–301.

4 Paediatric formulary committee (2009). *BNF for children*, 5th edn. Pharmaceutical Press, London.

5 Hetrick, S.E., Merry, S.N., McKenzie, J., Sindahl, P., and Proctor, M. (2007). Selective serotonin reuptake inhibitors (SSRIs) for depressive disorders in children and adolescents. *Cochrane Database Syst. Rev.* **2007** (3), CD004851.

6 Whittington, C.J., Kendall, T., Fonagy, P., Cottrell, D., Cotgrove, A., and Boddington, E. (2004). Selective serotonin reuptake inhibitors in childhood depression: systematic review of published versus unpublished data. *Lancet* **363** (9418), 1341–5.

7 Emslie, G.J., Kennard, B.D., Mayes, T.L., Nightingale-Teresi, J., Carmody, T., Hughes, C.W., *et al.* (2008). Fluoxetine versus placebo in preventing relapse of major depression in children and adolescents. *Am. J. Psychiatry* **165**, 459–67.

8 Hart, D. and Bossert, E. (1994). Self-reported fears of hospitalized school-age children. *J. Pediatr. Nurs.* **9** (2), 83–90.

9 Spinetta, J.J., Rigler, D., and Karon, M. (1973). Anxiety in the dying child. *Pediatrics* **52** (6), 841–5.

10 Ashton, H. (1994). Guidelines for the rational use of benzodiazepines. When and what to use. *Drugs* **48** (1), 25–40.

11 Birmaher, B., Axelson, D.A., Monk, K., Kalas, C., Clark, D.B., Ehmann, M., *et al.* (2003). Fluoxetine for the treatment of childhood anxiety disorders. *J. Am. Acad. Child Adolesc. Psychiatry* **42** (4), 415–23.

12 Jones, D.P. and Jones, E.A. (1963). Drugs for insomnia. *Can. Med. Assoc. J.* **89**, 1331.

13 Smits, M.G., van Stel, H.K., van der Heijden, K., Meijer, A.M., Coenen, A.M., and Kerkhof, G.A. (2003). Melatonin improves health status and sleep in children with idiopathic chronic sleep-onset insomnia: a randomized placebo-controlled trial. *J. Am. Acad. Child Adolesc. Psychiatry* **42** (11), 1286–93.

14 Zhdanova, I.V. (2005). Melatonin as a hypnotic: pro. *Sleep Med. Rev.* **9** (1), 51–65.

15 Breitbart, W. and Strout, D. (2000). Delirium in the terminally ill. *Clin. Geriatr. Med.* **16** (2), 357–72.

16 Breitbart, W., Marotta, R., Platt, M.M., Weisman, H., Deverenco, M., Grau, C., *et al.* (1996). A double-blind trial of haloperidol, chlorpromazine, and lorazepam in the treatment of delirium in hospitalized AIDS patients. *Am. J. Psychiatry* **153** (2), 231–7.

17 Stirling, L.C., Kurowska, A., and Tookman, A. (1999). The use of phenobarbitone in the management of agitation and seizures at the end of life. *J. Pain Symptom Manage.* **17** (5), 363–8.

# Skin symptoms

# Epidermolysis bullosa

**Definition** Epidermolysis bullosa is a rare (1 in 17 000 births) genetic condition that leads to fragile skin. It is characterized as a group of varying genetic disorders that produce blisters and shearing with minimal pressure or injury.

## General points
- Dependent on the type, children can have blisters anywhere on their skin or gastrointestinal tract.
- The lung, heart, and renal tract can all be involved.
- Many children have anaemia and malnutrition problems.
- There are 3 distinct types of epidermolysis bullosa (EB).[1]

## Epidermolysis bullosa simplex
- Most common type affecting 65–70% of all children with EB.
- Histologically shows lack of adhesion of the skin above the basement membrane.
- Inherited as dominant trait; often parents have a family history of condition (rarely due to gene mutation).
- Blisters affect hands and feet, although a rarer form can occur over the whole body.
- Most children will survive well into adulthood.
- Children can be born with severe blistering but it invariably improves with time.
- Made worse by heat.

## Junctional epidermolysis bullosa
- Most aggressive form affecting 5–10% of all children with EB.
- Histologically shows lack of adhesion of the skin through the basement membrane.
- Inherited recessively. Unexpected diagnosis for parents.
- Most serious type is the Herlitz form.
- 50% die within the first 2 years of life. The other 50% of children have a milder form and can do well.
- Children can develop severe systemic problems.
  - Gastrointestinal: blistering throughout the gastrointestinal tract making eating painful. Gastro-oesophageal reflux can lead to oesophageal strictures. Malnutrition with anaemia is common. Nasogastric tubes and gastrostomies can cause their own problems with the skin. Perianal blisters can cause pain on defecation and lead to constipation.
  - Anaemia: due to malnutrition and chronic blood loss from skin and mucosa.
  - Respiratory: bullae formation in the larynx leads to a hoarse cry and stridor.
  - Cardiac: rarely some children can develop fatal dilated cardiomyopathy.
  - Renal: occurs rarely.

## Dystrophic epidermolysis pullosa

- This type of EB derives its name from the fact that the blistering associated with the condition tends to heal with scar formation.
- Affects 25% of all children with EB.
- Children histologically show lack of adhesion of skin below the basement membrane.
- Can be inherited as dominant or recessive trait.
- There is wide variation in the severity of dystrophic EB.
- The mildest type (the dominant form) can allow an almost normal life. Unfortunately, this group has a high risk of developing squamous cell carcinoma of the skin before the age of 35 years. The average life expectancy after tumour diagnosis is 5 years.
- Most serious type is the recessive form known as Hallopeau–Siemens.
- Children with the more aggressive form of dystrophic EB can develop severe systemic problems similar to those of junctional EB. In addition children with dystrophic EB can also have problems with:
  - skin: scarring leads to severe contractures most notably to the hands;
  - gastrointestinal: scarring in the mouth can lead to the tongue becoming fused to the base of the mouth and subsequently loss of labial sulcus and microstomia; webs and strictures can form in the oesophagus;
  - renal: nephropathy and chronic post-infectious glomerulonephritis can occur.

# Managing epidermolysis bullosa

The management of EB requires a multidisciplinary approach organized and coordinated by specialized units. In the UK this would be via Great Ormond Street Hospital or Birmingham Children's Hospital.

- The first and foremost part of the management is to make the correct diagnosis by skin biopsy assessed by a unit specializing in this type of histopathology.
- Then the issues of handling, dressings, and symptom management need to be addressed.

## Handling

- Because skin will break down with minimal pressure or shearing force, handling should be kept to a minimum.
- Babies and small infants should be lifted using the roll and lift technique (rolled to one side and then one hand on the buttocks and the other on the head or neck).
- No children with EB should be lifted under their arms.
- Children should be cuddled gently as, due to hyperalgesia, children can experience pain from this.
- Children can be kissed gently.
- Older children may prefer to move themselves.
- Children with some types of EB can attend normal schools but there needs to be pre-planning in terms of teaching assistants, leaving classes early or late to avoid being bumped or knocked, etc.
- Bathing for some children may be impossible due to pain.

## Dressings

- Dressing changing can be a painful experience. This is due to pain from the skin lesions, hyperalgesia, and sometimes anticipatory pain.
- Correct non-adherent dressings should be used.
- Dressing changing should be kept to a minimum.
- Adequate analgesia should be used.
- Dressing changing should be done as quickly as possible as exposure of the wounds can be painful.

## Pain

- The management of pain follows the same principles as discussed in Chapters 5 to 8 but there are particular issues associated with procedural pain.[2]
- Non-pharmacological modalities such as physiotherapy and visualization can be very helpful.
- For mild pain from minor dressing changes, paracetamol or NSAIDs can be used.
- For more serve pain, entonox, fentanyl lozenges, or morphine given in sufficient time can be used.
- Anxiety may require a small dose of benzodiazepines such as lorazepam or midazolam.
- Background pain can be managed with slow release morphine.
- The neuropathic component of pain associated with EB responds well to amitriptyline or gabapentin.
- In the terminal phase a syringe driver can be used.

# Pruritus

**Definition** An unpleasant sensation that provokes a desire to scratch.

## Pathophysiology

- Arises in skin, conjunctivae, and mucous membranes.
- Can be classified as:[3]
  - cutaneous: arises from skin;
  - neuropathic: damage to nerves or by direct irritation;
  - psychological.
- Transmitted through C fibres (similar to pain).
- Receptors are more superficial than pain receptors.
- Fibres respond to pruritogens including histamine, acetylcholine, and peripheral serotonin.
- Pruritus increases with heat, anxiety, and boredom.

## Causes

- Opioids particularly can cause pruritus, and this is more common in children than adults.
- Drugs: many drugs can cause problems but particularly antibiotics (penicillin) and antiepileptics (phenytoin).
- Eczema or dry skin.
- Scabies or lice.
- Renal failure.
- Hepatic disease causing jaundice.
- Haematological disorders particularly leukaemias and lymphomas.
- AIDS.
- Psychological.

## Management

- Look at the possible causes and treat appropriately.
- Simple rehydration of the skin with moisturizers.
- Cut back nails with or without the use of mittens.
- Pruritus decreases with cold, distraction, and relaxation.
- Keep the child cool.
- Child should wear loose fitting cotton clothes.
- Calamine lotion.
- If the skin is inflamed then use mild steroid creams such as hydrocortisone.
- Oral corticosteroids can be used if the skin is very inflamed or for pruritus in terminal Hodgkin's lymphoma.
- NSAIDs can help by reducing prostaglandins, which can sensitize nerve endings to pruritogenic substances.
- $H_1$ antihistamines are used extensively in most types of pruritus but understanding the pathophysiology of pruritus clearly indicates that there will be occasions when they are poorly effective or completely ineffective.
- Serotonin antagonist (e.g. ondansetron) can relieve some types of opioid-induced[4] and cholestatic pruritus.

# Fungating tumours

### General points

- Fungating tumours are rare in children.
- Fungating tumours occur when a primary or secondary tumour invades through the skin leading to breakdown and ulceration of the skin.
- The tumour may spread locally or break down into a cavity.
- The resulting necrosis of the tissue may then become infected, bleed, or discharge exudate.
- In children the issues around disfigurement, body image, and smell may cause considerable psychological problems.

### Causes

- Rhabdomyosarcoma.
- Nerve sheath tumours (e.g. complicating neurofibromatosis).
- Squamous cell carcinoma.
- Lymphoma.

### Management

- Treat reversible factors:
  - improve nutrition;
  - stop or reduce steroids.
- Modify the appearance of the tumour:
  - surgery by debulking;
  - radiotherapy;
  - chemotherapy.
- Control pain:
  - during dressing changes consider entonox, fentanyl lozenge, oral morphine;
  - localized pain: consider topical diamorphine soaked into a dressing or topical anaesthetic agents such as lidocaine;
  - chronic pain: use slow release morphine.
- Exudates:
  - use appropriate dressings (Chapter 15, Managing pressure sores, Table 15.1 p. 173).
- Odour:
  - a counter-odour, e.g. household air freshener or aromatherapy oils;
  - a deodorant, e.g. ostomy deodorizers or electric deodorizer;
  - metronidazole either topically or systemically to treat anaerobic organisms;
  - live yoghurt;
  - charcoal impregnated dressings;
  - occlusive dressings either OpSite® (total) or Granuflex® (almost total);
  - honey and icing sugar dressings.
- If haemorrhage is a problem:
  - topical adrenaline 1 in 1000;
  - calcium alginate dressings have haemostatic properties;
  - radiotherapy;
  - use non-adherent dressings and soak off with normal saline.
- If surrounding skin at risk from exudate:
  - protect with barrier ointment.

# Pressure sores

## General points

This is one symptom in which there is universal agreement with the old adage 'prevention is better than cure'.

- Continual assessment of the skin is essential in all children with life-limiting conditions. This should not be just a nursing duty but should be part of the regular medical check of all children by doctors.
- Paediatric nurses often have very limited experience of managing pressure sores. It is often helpful to involve specialist wound care nurses from the adult world as the principles of treatment are the same.
- It is important to make dressings cosmetically acceptable to the child.
- Try to remove dressings with minimal pain.
- Try to lengthen the time between dressing changes.
- Cost-effectiveness of the different types of dressings should be appreciated.
- The Braden Q Scale for assessing risk of pressure sores in the paediatric population is the best validated of all the scales, but even this scale is not completely accurate for children in the acute hospital setting.[5,6]

## Risk factors

The risk factors associated with developing pressure sores are:[7]

- tissue ischaemia by external pressure sufficient to overcome capillary pressure;
- sensory perception;
- skin moisture;
- activity;
- mobility;
- risk of friction and shear;
- nutritional status;
- incontinence.

## Staging

A staging system has been devised and is helpful in the management of pressure sores:[8]

- stage 1: intact skin but erythema present;
- stage 2: partial skin damage to epidermis and dermis;
- stage 3: full thickness damage down to subcutaneous tissue;
- stage 4: extensive damage down to underlying structures such as muscle or tendon.

# Managing pressure sores

- Prevention with early aggressive intervention.
- Monitor pressure points.
- Regular turning.
- Pressure-relieving measures:
  - appropriate mattresses, air beds being the best;
  - sheepskin bedding;
  - pressure-relieving cushions.
- Assess and manage the child's nutritional status. Dietitians are particularly useful.
- Maintain good skin care with good hygiene and hydration.

Table 15.1 lists the types of dressings and their uses.
- For stage 1 pressure sore:
  - use occlusive dressing/films to protect the sore;
  - be careful when removing not to cause further traumatic damage to surrounding skin.
- For healing ulcers undergoing epithelialization:
  - film dressings;
  - low adherent dressings;
  - hydrocolloid interactive dressings.
- For light exudate:
  - film dressings;
  - hydrocolloid interactive dressings;
  - low adherent dressings;
  - alginate dressings;
  - hydrophilic foam dressings.
- For heavy exudate:
  - hydrocolloid interactive dressings;
  - hydrogel with secondary dressings;
  - alginate dressings;
  - hydrophilic foam dressings;
  - use of paediatric stoma bag.
- For cavities:
  - alginate cavity dressing;
  - silastic foam if wound is clean;
  - foam dressing.
- If debridement is required:
  - surgery;
  - enzymes;
  - hydrocolloid paste with dressing;
  - hydrogel.
- If the wound is infected:
  - topical metronidazole;
  - irrigate wound with iv metronidazole solution;
  - systemic antibiotics;
  - honey and icing sugar dressings.

**Table 15.1** Types of dressing and their uses[9]

| Type | Common names | Notes |
| --- | --- | --- |
| Films | OpSite®, Tegaderm® | Allow observation; cannot absorb exudate |
| Low adherent | Release®, Mepore® | Absorbs some exudate |
| Hydrocolloids | Granuflex®, Comfeel®, DuoDerm® | May be left for up to 1 week |
| Hydrogels | IntraSite® Gel, Iodosorb® | Absorb large amounts of exudate |
| Alginates | Kaltostat®, Sorbsan® | Haemostatic |
| Foams | Lyofoam®, Silastic® | For cavities |

## References

**1** Fine, J.D., Eady, R.A., Bauer, E.A., Briggaman, R.A., Bruckner-Tuderman, L., Christiano, A., *et al.* (2000). Revised classification system for inherited epidermolysis bullosa: Report of the Second International Consensus Meeting on diagnosis and classification of epidermolysis bullosa. *J. Am. Acad. Dermatol.* **42** (6), 1051–66.

**2** Herod, J., Denyer, J., Goldman, A., and Howard, R. (2002). Epidermolysis bullosa in children: pathophysiology, anaesthesia and pain management. *Paediatr. Anaesth.* **12** (5), 388–97.

**3** Twycross, R., Greaves, M.W., Handwerker, H., Jones, E.A., Libretto, S.E., Szpietowski, J.C., and Zylicz, Z. (2003). Itch: scratching more than the surface. *Q. J. Med.* **96** (1), 7–26.

**4** Kyriakides, K., Hussain, S.K., and Hobbs, G.J. (1999). Management of opioid-induced pruritus: a role for 5-HT3 antagonists? *Br. J. Anaesth.* **82** (3), 439–41.

**5** Quigley, S.M. and Curley, M.A. (1996). Skin integrity in the pediatric population: preventing and managing pressure ulcers. *J. Soc. Pediatr. Nurs.* **1** (1), 7–18.

**6** Pallija, G., Mondozzi, M., and Webb, A.A. (1999). Skin care of the pediatric patient. *J. Pediatr. Nurs.* **14** (2), 80–7.

**7** Bergstrom, N., Braden, B.J., Laguzza, A., and Holman, V. (1987). The Braden scale for predicting pressure sore risk. *Nurs. Res.* **36** (4), 205–10.

**8** National Pressure Ulcer Advisory Panel (1992). *Statement on pressure ulcer prevention*, Agency for Health Care Policy and Research, Reston, Virginia.. Available at ℅ http://www.npuap.org/positn1.htm

**9** Twycross, R.G. and Wilcock, A. (2001). *Symptom management in advanced cancer*, 3rd edn. Radcliffe Medical Press, Abingdon.

# Palliative care emergencies

# Introduction

Emergencies are relatively rare in paediatric palliative medicine. They can be defined as 'situations needing pre-planning'.

The key principles to managing palliative care emergencies are the following.
- Anticipate that they may happen.
- Recognize early that they are happening.
- Have a plan ready for when they do happen.

Paediatric palliative medicine emergencies should always be managed by the tertiary paediatric palliative medicine team where one is available, or in collaboration with a specialist adult palliative medicine team otherwise.

There are six emergencies:
- cord compression;
- catastrophic haemorrhage;
- severe uncontrolled pain;
- superior vena cava obstruction;
- intestinal obstruction;
- hypercalcaemia.

# Cord compression

### Pathophysiology
- Usually a complication of cancer.
- Can occur as a result of soft tissue expansion or sudden vertebral collapse.
- In children, acute cord compression rare.

### Signs and symptoms
- Classically, sudden onset of back pain.
- Neurological symptoms, particularly loss of bladder or bowel control.
- Sudden and unexplained lack of mobility.
- In children, onset typically more insidious than in adults and classic symptoms and signs may not appear.

### Management
- Depends on situation.
- Reduction of tumour oedema through high dose dexamethasone.
- Reduction of tumour mass through radiation or emergency debulking surgery.
- Outcome for neurological recovery is poor if symptoms have been present for more than 48h.
- In practice, cord compression in children is typically non-acute, and it is rare for neurological recovery to be possible in the palliative situation.
- Invasive interventions such as surgery are usually not appropriate in children.

# Catastrophic haemorrhage

### Pathophysiology

- Usually complicates tumours close to or eroding through a major vessel.
- In reality very rare.
- Greatly feared by families and patients.

### Signs and symptoms

- May complicate lymphopoietic conditions such as leukaemia in which platelet numbers and function are both reduced.
- Often preceded by oozing, epistaxis, or haemoptysis.
- Correlation of platelet numbers with risk of haemorrhage is poor, and platelet numbers alone should not be an indication for transfusion.

### Management

- Be aware of possibility and anticipate it.
- Platelet transfusions, tranexamic acid, etamsylate to optimize clotting.
- Soften impact by discussion with family, and provision of green towels against which blood is less obvious should haemorrhage occur.
- Arrange for parenteral quick acting anxiolytic such as midazolam, and analgesics such as diamorphine to be by the patient's bedside in case haemorrhage should occur.

# Severe uncontrolled pain

## Pathophysiology
- Rare in paediatric palliative medicine.
- Often results from inexpert opioid titration and adjuvant prescription in early stages of pain.
- Always has major anxiety and fear component.

## Signs and symptoms
- Pain suddenly becoming worse, often with no obvious cause.
- Apparent ineffectiveness even of large doses of opioids.

## Management
- Involve specialist palliative care team as soon as diagnosis is made.
- Use parenteral route to secure control as soon as possible.
- Palliative care team will administer slow injection of opioid until pain goes.
- Calculation of regular and breakthrough opioid dose is made on basis of dose required to control pain.

# Superior vena cava obstruction

### Pathophysiology
- Venous obstruction in the mediastinum and upper chest.
- Usual cause is tumour, particularly lymphoma.
- Pulmonary congestion leads to dyspnoea.
- Congestion of intracranial vessels leads to feeling of fullness and headache.

### Signs and symptoms
- Headache, pressure, or 'fullness' in head, worse on sneezing or bending forwards.
- Shortness of breath and discomfort in chest.
- Facial plethora, obvious collateral vessels over the upper chest wall.

### Management
- Management of individual symptoms (particularly pain and dyspnoea).
- Reduction of tumour oedema using steroids (▶ use in discussion with oncologists as some lymphomas may be very sensitive to steroids).
- Reduction of tumour mass using radiotherapy.
- Surgical insertion of stent into the SVC.

# Intestinal obstruction

## Pathophysiology
- Obstruction leads to proximal dilatation.
- Dilatation leads to stretching of gut wall.
- Stretching of gut wall leads to increased secretion.
- Increase secretion exacerbates dilatation.
- Relatively rare in children.
- May occur with abdominal tumours such as neuroblastoma or where there is abdominal extension of pelvic tumours.

## Signs and symptoms
- Nausea and vomiting.
- Constipation.
- Severe intermittent colicky abdominal pain.
- Abdominal dilatation.
- Usually occurring in context of known abdominal tumour.

## Management
- Surgery sometimes an option if single discrete obstruction
- Reduce spasm (anticholinergics, e.g. hyoscine hydrobromide).
- Strong analgesia (e.g. diamorphine).
- Antiemetics (e.g. haloperidol).
- Reduce secretions (reduce fluid intake, nil by mouth, consider octreotide).
- Consider prokinetics (e.g. metoclopromide) if obstruction is not complete, such that there is the possibility of spontaneous resolution.
- Consider steroids to reduce tumour oedema.

▶ Prokinetics and anticholinergics are mutually inhibitory and should not usually be used together. As many as half of all intestinal obstruction associated with malignant disease may resolve spontaneously without the need for surgical intervention.

# Hypercalcaemia

### Pathophysiology
- Extremely rare in children, as associated with adult cancers such as breast, thyroid, and prostate.
- May occur in context of extensive metastatic bone disease or hormone-secreting tumours.

### Signs and symptoms
- Severe and intolerable symptoms: must be treated urgently.
- Pain (bone and abdominal).
- Nausea and vomiting.
- Confusion.
- Diuresis

### Management
- Involve specialist palliative care team early.
- Treat underlying cause if possible (radiotherapy to multiple lytic lesions caused by leukaemia).
- Parenteral fluids.
- Diuretics.
- Bisphosphonate therapy (parenteral and oral for maintenance).

## Summary

Whilst it is true that emergencies are rare in paediatric palliative medicine, they can cause considerable fear and suffering. To pre-empt this, those working with children with life-limiting conditions should anticipate the possibility of an emergency, recognize it early, and have a plan ready.

Management of palliative medicine emergencies always requires the involvement of tertiary services. Ideally, this should be a paediatric palliative medicine service, but where none is available, advice should urgently be sought from the adult palliative medicine team locally.

# Malignant diseases

# Introduction

Cancer in childhood is a group of heterogeneous conditions linked largely by their pathogenesis. There are several reviews of symptoms occurring in childhood cancer.[1–3] The symptoms a child will experience depend on:

- the particular diagnosis;
- its primary location;
- the pattern of spread;
- the extent and nature of prior treatment;
- its secondary consequences (e.g. bone marrow suppression).

With respect to palliative medicine, malignant diseases can be considered in three broad groups:

- haemopoietic malignancies (leukaemia and lymphoma);
- central nervous system tumours (usually brain);
- other solid tumours.

The likelihood of needing referral for specialist palliative medicine is clearly governed by prognosis as well as incidence:[1]

- 39% of referrals are for solid tumours (excluding CNS);
- 36% of referrals are for CNS tumours;
- 25% of referrals are for haemopoietic malignancies.

## CNS tumours

- Astrocytomas.
- Medulloblastoma.
- Ependymoma.
- Brainstem glioma.

## Haemopoietic malignancies

- Acute myeloid leukaemia.
- Acute lymphoid leukaemia.
- Hodgkin's lymphoma.
- Non-Hodgkin's lymphoma.
- Chronic leukaemias (rare).

## Other solid tumours:

- Rhabdomyosarcoma.
- Neuroblastoma.
- Osteosarcoma.
- Ewing's sarcoma.
- Wilms' tumour.
- Other sarcomas.

# Symptoms in cancer

Most of what follows comes from a single study.[1] The 10 commonest symptoms experienced by children with cancer are:

- pain (92%);
- weakness (91%);
- anorexia (68%);
- weight loss (67%);
- mobility (61%);
- nausea or vomiting (59%);
- constipation (59%);
- sleep disturbance (49%);
- anxiety and depression (45%);
- dyspnoea (40%).

However, these symptoms are not experienced by all three groups equally.

- Top five symptoms in non-CNS solid tumours:
  - pain (98%);
  - weakness (94%);
  - weight loss (88%);
  - anorexia (84%);
  - constipation (67%).
- Top five symptoms experienced by those with CNS tumours:
  - weakness (93%);
  - mobility problems (89%);
  - pain (81%);
  - difficulties with speech (76%);
  - excess secretions (70%).
- Top five symptoms experienced by children with haemopoietic malignancies (leukaemia or lymphoma):
  - pain (95%);
  - weakness (83%);
  - bleeding (66%);
  - infection (59%);
  - anorexia and weight loss (56%).

Despite palliative care, there is a tendency for symptoms to become more frequent and more severe as death approaches. This is particularly marked for symptoms for which there are few effective interventions available, such as:

- weakness;
- weight loss;
- swallowing, excess secretions;
- sleep disturbance.

▶ These are also the symptoms experienced by children with CNS tumours, making palliative care in this group particularly challenging.

# Managing symptoms in paediatric oncology

- The palliative care team should ideally be familiar to the family before curative treatment is discontinued.
- Palliative management and potentially curative management can, and often should, proceed simultaneously.
- Palliative chemotherapy and radiotherapy should be considered in collaboration with the oncology team.
- Most tertiary oncology teams will include paediatric oncology outreach nurse specialists who may also be experienced and/or trained in paediatric palliative care.

## The role of chemotherapy once cure is no longer expected

Even once it is acknowledged that there is no prospect of cure, chemotherapy may continue to be prescribed for one or more of the following reasons:[4]

- as part of a clinical trial;
- to 'buy time' for the child;
- at the request of family who feel that everything should be done;
- to relieve symptoms—in effect, as an adjuvant.

Chemotherapy is often called 'palliative' in any of these situations, but the term should properly be reserved only for the last. 'Palliative' indicates that its intent is primarily to relieve symptoms.

With respect to the use of chemotherapy when cure is no longer expected, the following points should be considered.

- The benefit must always outweigh the burden.
- Delaying death should do more than simply prolong dying.
- It is not appropriate to prescribe chemotherapy at the request of the family, unless it is in the child's own best interest to do so.
- Many young people value the opportunity to take part in clinical trials for altruistic reasons. The principle of equipoise means it is not expected that such trials will benefit them and this should be made clear.
- Many chemotherapy agents are relatively non-toxic and can provide significant symptom relief if properly used (e.g. vincristine, oral etoposide, oral 6-mercaptopurine). In this context, chemotherapy is, in effect, acting as an adjuvant to analgesia. *This is the only correct use of the term 'palliative chemotherapy' since its purpose is to relieve symptoms without influencing disease course.*

## References

**1** Goldman, A., Hewitt, M., Collins, G.S., Childs, M., and Hain, R. (2006). Symptoms in children/ young people with progressive malignant disease: United Kingdom Children's Cancer Study Group/Paediatric Oncology Nurses Forum survey. *Pediatrics* **117** (6), e1179–86.

**2** Hongo, T., Watanabe, C., Okada, S., Inoue, N., Yajima, S., Fujii, Y., *et al.* (2003). Analysis of the circumstances at the end of life in children with cancer: symptoms, suffering and acceptance. *Pediatr. Int.* **45** (1), 60–4.

**3** Wolfe, J., Grier, H.E., Klar, N., Levin, S.B., Ellenbogen, J.M., Salem-Schatz, S., *et al.* (2000). Symptoms and suffering at the end of life in children with cancer [see comments]. *N. Engl. J. Med.* **342** (5), 326–33.

**4** Hain, R., Maisey, K., Cox, R., Kus, T., Devins, M., and Davies, R. (2004). Ethical dimensions of palliative chemotherapy. *Arch. Dis. Child.* **89** (S1), A35.

# Specific non-malignant diseases

# Introduction

The cross-section of life-limiting conditions affecting children is quite different from those in adults. In adult palliative care, the vast majority of work is around malignant conditions, whilst in paediatric palliative care the work is based equally on malignant and non-malignant conditions.

The number of life-limiting conditions in paediatrics is vast; the Contact a Family (CaF) directory of specific conditions and rare disorders (℘ www.cafamily.org.uk) holds details of over 1000 different conditions. In view of this number it is almost impossible for any one doctor to know the details of all the conditions.

In the authors' opinion, it is best to have a good working knowledge of the most common non-malignant disorders and then obtain the details of other rarer conditions as required. In many cases of the rarer disorders, little may be known about the trajectory of the condition. In other cases that are seen, we may not even have a diagnosis and so have no idea what to expect from the illness. Fortunately, an empirical approach to assessment and management of illness is very effective in such situations.

There are several medical conditions that are common enough for it to be helpful to know about them in more detail. As all the conditions by definition have no cure it is best to tackle each symptom the child presents with individually, never forgetting that medical intervention is not the only modality open to us. The full array of the multidisciplinary team is required to effect the best holistic care. This is discussed in length in the Duchenne muscular dystrophy section but the same principles need to be carried through with regard to other conditions.

# Duchenne muscular dystrophy

Duchenne muscular dystrophy (DMD) is the second most common single-gene disorder in Western countries.

## Genetics

- DMD is caused by a gene defect on the X chromosome at the Xp21 level. This gene produces a very large protein called dystrophin. This is present in very small amounts in normal muscle but is virtually absent or nonfunctional in the muscles of patients with DMD.
- Dystrophin combines with a glycoprotein to form a complex that is essential for muscle cell membrane. Disruption of the complex leads to muscle cell death.
- DMD is inherited as an X-linked recessive trait. The mutant gene is always fully penetrant.

## Diagnosis

Diagnosis is confirmed with the triad of tests:
- serum creatine kinase (50–100 times normal);
- muscle biopsy;
- DNA analysis.

## Clinical features[1]

- The onset is slow and average age of diagnosis is 5 years (can be as late as 8–9 years)
- Early symptoms are delay in walking, tip toeing, recurrent falls, and inability to run.
- Early signs are:
  - inability to run;
  - inability to stand on one leg (positive Trendelenburg);
  - inability to lift their head off the bed;
  - inability to rise from sitting with folded arms; the child uses his arms to climb up his thighs (Gowers' manoeuvre);
  - sliding through the examiner's hands when lifted from under the arms.
- Progression is seen over time as:
  - lumbar lordosis;
  - waddling gait;
  - equinovarus deformity from shortening of the Achilles tendon;
  - 95% of the boys become wheelchair bound by the age of 12 years The earlier the child becomes wheelchair bound the poorer the prognosis.
- Late stage signs:
  - contractures of other tendons;
  - severe kyphoscoliosis;
  - weakness of the intercostal muscles;
  - respiratory problems with hypoventilation and hypercapnia at night;
  - patients with diurnal hypercapnia will die within 9.7 months (mean value) without ventilation;
  - respiratory failure with infection is the commonest cause of death.

*Other organ system involvement*
Although the skeletal muscle is the main tissue involved in DMD, other tissues and organs can be affected. These complications occur in only some of the children.

- Cardiac muscle:
  - involvement can lead to arrhythmia, and heart failure;
  - 15% of DMD cases die of primary cardiomyopathy.
- Gastrointestinal:
  - constipation;
  - paralytic ileus;
  - gastric dilatation,
- Bladder:
  - rarely bladder paralysis.
- Vascular:
  - increased bleeding tendency noted after spinal surgery;
  - poor circulation.
- Central nervous system:
  - lowered IQ to 80 average.
- Skeletal system (secondary to immobility rather than disease):
  - impaired development of major bones;
  - skeletal deformity;
  - osteoporosis.

# Management and prognosis for Duchenne muscular dystrophy

## Management

Management for any incurable disease is linked to improving quality of life and increasing survival by working with a multidisciplinary team.
- Specialist neurodisability units:
  - to supply expert advice;
  - coordinate appropriate care.
- Community and hospital paediatricians:
  - day to day medical care;
  - to control symptoms.
- Palliative care team:
  - to control difficult symptoms.
- Dietitian:
  - to improve nutrition and weight control.
- Physiotherapy:
  - to maintain ambulation as long as possible;
  - to stretch muscles and tendons and hence reduce severity of contractures, including teaching the parents;
  - to advise on the right forms of splints and walking aids;
  - to advise on wheelchairs, posture, and support.
- Occupational therapist.
- Surgeon:
  - for release of contractures;
  - to correct spinal deformity;
  - to help with the high fracture rate (up to 20%).
- Cardiologist:
  - to monitor and treat all the cardiac symptoms.
- Respiratory physician:
  - to monitor respiratory function and plan best time for ventilation;
  - treatment of respiratory infection;
  - vaccinations.
- Home ventilation team:
  - to help the child and family learn about, use, and maintain the most appropriate ventilation system.
- Psychologist.
- Educational team.
- Social services.

**Prognosis** The prognosis of DMD has continued to improve over the last four decades (Table 18.1). Each improvement, however, as with any incurable disease, leads to new problems that have to be faced by the patient, family, and health care professionals.

**Table 18.1** Mean age of survival over time in a patient with DMD[2]

| Decade | Mean age of survival (years) |
| --- | --- |
| 1960s | 14.3 |
| 1980s (with better medical care) | 19 |
| 2000s (with ventilation) | 24.3 |

# Mucopolysaccharidoses

The mucopolysaccharide (MPS) illnesses are all genetic lysosomal storage conditions. Mucopolysaccharides are now called glycosaminoglycans (GAG). In the various conditions there is a genetic abnormality that prevents or significantly reduces the production of specific enzymes. As a result the body is unable to break down certain waste products. These products cannot be excreted by the body and so are stored within the lysosomes of cells throughout the body, causing damage to a wide range of tissues. The conditions caused are not apparent at birth but soon develop over time as the storage of material increases. There is a range of conditions but here we will discuss the three most common types.

# MPS type 1, (Hurler's syndrome)[3]

- There are 3 subsets of conditions classified as MPS 1. Of these Hurler's is the most severe.
- Hurler's syndrome is caused by a lack of an enzyme called lysosomal alpha-L-iduronidase.
- It is caused by a recessive gene.

*Clinical features*
- Facial changes can be seen from 2 years of age.
- Most symptoms develop between ages 3 and 8 years.
- Growth retardation from age 3 years.
- Coarse facial features with:
  - short nose;
  - low nose bridge;
  - flat facies;
  - large head;
  - tongue is enlarged and may stick out;
  - thick lips.
- Corneal clouding.
- Deafness.
- Musculoskeletal:
  - bent over posture when walking;
  - scoliosis;
  - joint disease with stiffness;
  - claw hand;
  - nerve entrapment including carpal tunnel syndrome.
- Mental retardation dependent on severity of condition.
- Respiratory problems secondary to:
  - runny nose;
  - enlarged tonsils and adenoids;
  - chest wall deformity;
  - pressure on the diaphragm from enlarged liver and spleen;
  - sleep apnoea;
  - recurrent chest infections.
- Cardiac problems:
  - cardiomyopathy;
  - endocardiofibroelastosis;
  - coronary heart disease;
  - aortic and mitral valve disease.
- Gastrointestinal:
  - protruding belly;
  - hepatosplenomegaly;
  - umbilical and inguinal herniae;
  - diarrhoea and constipation.

*Prognosis* As there is a range of severity associated with MPS type 1, with Hurler's being the most severe, the prognosis is also variable. In the most severe cases the child is likely to die before their teenage years; in the mildest form the child may live into young adulthood.

# MPS type 2, (Hunter's syndrome)[4]

- Hunter's syndrome is caused by a lack of an enzyme called iduronate sulfatase.
- It is an X-linked recessive genetic disorder.
- Originally thought of as two separate types, juvenile onset and late onset, but now thought to be a spectrum with the two subsets just being extremes on the scale.

### Clinical features

As per MPS type 1 but with these additional features:

- mental retardation dependent on severity of condition;
- aggressive behaviour;
- hyperactivity.

**Prognosis** In the most severe cases child is likely to die aged 10–20 years. In the mildest form patient may live up to 50 or 60 years of age.

# Mucopolysaccharidosis type 3 (Sanfilippo syndrome)

- MPS 3[5] is possibly the most common type of MPS.
- There are 4 types of Sanfilippo syndrome characterized by 4 different enzyme deficiencies:
  - type A: an enzyme called heparan N-sulfatase;
  - type B: an enzyme called alpha-N-acetylglucosaminidase;
  - type C: an enzyme called acetyl-CoAlpha-glucosaminide acetyltransferase;
  - type D: an enzyme called N-acetylglucosamine 6-sulfatase.
- Clinically all four types are the same.
- It is an autosomal recessive disorder.

*Clinical features*
- MPS type 3 has all the features seen in MPS types 1 and 2 but generally to a much milder level.
- Because the glycosaminoglycan that these four enzymes break down is primarily found in the CNS, the main clinical problems that are seen relate to its effect on the brain:
  - hyperactivity;
  - restlessness;
  - behavioural problems—often severe;
  - insomnia;
  - severe mental retardation;
  - unsteadiness;
  - recurrent falls;
  - loss of ambulation; some become wheelchair bound;
  - muscle spasms;
  - dystonia;
  - seizures both grand and petit mal;
  - difficulty swallowing;
  - chewing of fingers and clothes.

**Prognosis** In the most severe cases the child is likely to die aged 10–20 years. In the mildest form the patient may live up to 30 years of age.

# Batten's disease

- Batten's disease is part of a range of rare conditions known as neuronal ceroid lipofuscinoses (or NCLs).
- Batten's disease originally was described as the juvenile form of NCLs but now the name appears to encompass all the various types.
- There are four main types of NCL: infantile, late infantile, juvenile, and adult.[6] Each becomes apparent and progresses differently.
- NCLs involve a build up of an abnormal material called lipofuscin in the brain, probably due to an inability to remove or recycle protein by the brain. This same problem can occur in the eye, skin, muscle, and other tissues.
- It is an autosomal recessive disorder.

## Clinical features of juvenile NCL (Batten's disease)[7]

- Onset between 4 and 10 years of age (mean of 5 years).
- Visual loss.
- Speech disorder.
- Epilepsy of various types.
- Myoclonus.
- Mental retardation can be very severe.
- Movement disorder.
- Behavioural problems.
- Extrapyramidal signs with unsteady gait and ataxia.
- Sleep disturbance.

**Prognosis** In the most severe cases the child is likely to die in their late teens. In the milder form the patient may live up to 30 years of age.

# Spinal muscular atrophy

- Spinal muscular atrophy (SMA) is the second leading cause of neuromuscular disease.
- It is characterized by progressive muscle weakness due to degeneration of nerve cells in the anterior horn of the spinal tract and the brainstem nuclei.
- There are various subtypes but it now appears that these are all part of a continuum of disease expression related to the genetic disorder.
- It is an autosomal recessive disorder.

## Clinical features[8,9]

- Onset:
  - SMA type 1 within 6 months of birth;
  - SMA type 2, 6–12 months of age;
  - SMA type 3, after 12 months of age.
- SMA type 1:
  - weakness at birth;
  - poor muscle tone;
  - muscle weakness;
  - lack of motor development;
  - mild contractures;
  - absence of tendon reflex;
  - lack of head control;
  - feeding difficulties;
  - breathing difficulties;
  - muscle fasciculations.
- SMA type 2:
  - less severe than type 1;
  - progressive weakness;
  - poor posture.
- SMA type 3:
  - least severe;
  - affects shoulder muscle and proximal muscle first;
  - progressive weakness.

## Prognosis[10,11]

- Death within:
  - SMA type 1 less than 2–3 years;
  - SMA type 2 early infancy;
  - SMA type 3 within childhood.

# Trisomy 18 (Edward's syndrome)

Trisomy 18 is a genetic chromosomal condition where there is extra material within chromosome 18. It is relatively common, affecting girls three times more than boys.

## Clinical features
- Low birth weight.
- Growth retardation.
- Physical appearance:
  - microcephaly;
  - micrognathia;
  - chest wall abnormality;
  - low set ears;
  - clenched hands;
  - crossed legs.
- Neurological:
  - mental retardation;
  - seizures;
  - increased muscle tone.
- Cardiac:
  - congential heart defects;
  - ventricular septal defect;
  - atrial septal defect;
  - patent ductus arteriosus;
  - valve defects.
- Renal:
  - polycystic kidneys;
  - hydronephrosis.
- Coloboma.
- Diastasis recti.
- Hernias:
  - umbilical;
  - inguinal.
- Undescended testes.
- Defects of hands and feet.

## Prognosis[12]
- 50% of all affected babies die within the first week of life.
- 95% of all affected babies die within 1 year.

## References

**1** Emery, A. and Muntoni, F. (2004). *Duchenne muscular dystrophy*, 3rd edn. Oxford University Press, Oxford.

**2** Eagle, M., Baudouin, S.V., Chandler, C., Giddings, D.R., Bullock, R., and Bushby, K. (2002). Survival in Duchenne muscular dystrophy: improvements in life expectancy since 1967 and the impact of home nocturnal ventilation. *Neuromuscul. Disord.* **12** (10), 926–9.

**3** The National MPS Society (2008). *A guide to understanding MPS I*. The National MPS Society, Durham, North Carolina.

**4** The National MPS Society (2008). *A guide to understanding MPS II*. The National MPS Society, Durham, North Carolina.

**5** The National MPS Society (2008). *A guide to understanding MPS III*. The National MPS Society, Durham, North Carolina.

**6** Wisniewski, K.E., Zhong, N., and Philippart, M. (2001). Pheno/genotypic correlations of neuronal ceroid lipofuscinoses. *Neurology* **57** (4), 576–81.

**7** Backman, M.L., Santavuori, P.R., Aberg, L.E., and Aronen, E.T. (2005). Psychiatric symptoms of children and adolescents with juvenile neuronal ceroid lipofuscinosis. *J. Intellect. Disabil. Res.* **49** (Pt, 1), 25–32.

**8** Moosa, A. and Dubowitz, V. (1973). Spinal muscular atrophy in childhood. Two clues to clinical diagnosis. *Arch. Dis. Child.* **48** (5), 386–8.

**9** Iannaccone, S.T., Browne, R.H., Samaha, F.J., Buncher, C.R., and DCN/SMA Group (1993). Prospective study of spinal muscular atrophy before age 6 years. *Pediatr. Neurol.* **9** (3), 187–93.

**10** Ignatius, J. (1994). The natural history of severe spinal muscular atrophy—further evidence for clinical subtypes. *Neuromuscul. Disord.* **4** (5–6), 527–8.

**11** Russman, B.S., Buncher, C.R., White, M., Samaha, F.J., Iannaccone, S.T., and DCN/SMA Group (1996). Function changes in spinal muscular atrophy II and III. The DCN/SMA Group. *Neurology* **47** (4), 973–6.

**12** Rasmussen, S.A., Wong, L.Y., Yang, Q., May, K.M., and Friedman, J.M. (2003). Population-based analyses of mortality in trisomy 13 and trisomy 18. *Pediatrics* **111** (4 Pt 1), 777–84.

# Practicalities around time of death

# Introduction

There are different types of paediatric deaths:
1 sudden unexpected death;
2 a child with a life-limiting condition who dies unexpectedly;
3 a child with a life-limiting condition who has an expected death.

For the purpose of this chapter we will be discussing points 2 and 3 but health care professionals dealing with a situation in point 1 may still find much of the information useful.

In helping children to have a 'good death' it is vitally important to understand the practical issues around death. Parents often have little or no understanding of this and will look to the health care professional for guidance. When done well the parents are left unaware of the complexities involved. However, when done badly, the parents can be left feeling very upset.

The legal aspects to death in this chapter pertain to UK law.[1] Readers in other countries should make themselves familiar with the law of the country in which they are practising.

# Predictors of death

Predicting the time of death for a child is notoriously difficult.[2] Experience has taught us that we are frequently having to tell parents that their child is about to die, only for the child to recover and be discharged home. Sadly this is only temporary and child then presents again days, weeks, or months later. This emotional rollercoaster is very draining for the parents Therefore, the parents should be advised to take each day as it comes.

In some situations we can as health care professional anticipate that a child's condition may continue to deteriorate on to death:

- certain malignancies such as brain tumours;
- malignancies where all forms of treatment have failed and disease progression is seen as rapid;
- when specific organ failure is occurring such as liver or renal failure and the rate is documented as progressive;
- a child starts to have increasingly prolonged periods of sleep apnoea;
- seizure frequency and intensity continue to increase to a level where the seizures and the treatment for them begin to lead to secondary infection or respiratory suppression;
- Cheyne–Stokes breathing occurs.

# Before death

When we know that death is inevitable certain actions can be taken to help the situation.

- Check with the parents regarding their wishes (this may take many conversations).
- Check with the child if they are able to communicate.
- Follow any advanced directive protocol (individual or regional).
- All unnecessary drugs should be stopped.
- All unnecessary tubes, lines, and monitors should be removed.
- A PRP (personal resuscitation plan) should be discussed and recorded.
- In the hospice clear instruction regarding the parents' wishes should be documented in the notes.
- At home the ambulance service should be notified not to resuscitate and clear instruction to the out of hours services should be logged on to their computer system.
- Allow family and friends unlimited access to the child (subject to the child and parents not being overwhelmed).
- Call whichever religious leader the family request.
- Allow the family to approach the death of their child in the way they think best (some children have passed away listening to their favourite music, having early birthday or Christmas parties, or even dying peacefully in their bed but outside in the garden).

# Certifying and registering a death

When a child dies the parents will often turn to the health care professional for confirmation of death.

- At this stage the doctor should be called.
- Suitably trained nurses can 'verify' death but only doctors may 'certify' death for legal purposes.
- To verify/certify death check the following:
  - feel for carotid or femoral pulse for 1 full minute;
  - listen for breath sounds and observe rise and fall of chest for 1 full minute;
  - examine the eyes for pupil reaction using a torch. Pupils should be fixed and dilated.
- Inform the family/next of kin that death has taken place.

At this stage the doctor needs to ascertain as to whether the death needs to be referred to the coroner (see Chapter 19, Coroner, p. 216).

If the death was expected (and not a coroner's case) then
- the doctor should issue a death certificate (see box);
- the family can call their funeral director;
- the funeral director will give detailed information to the family regarding the processes involved for the funeral;
- the body can be kept at home or transferred to the funeral director's offices;
- within a hospice the body can be moved to the 'special room';
- the child's key worker should arrange for all the health care professionals involved with the child to be notified of the death.

## Registrar of births and deaths

- All deaths have to be registered by the registrar of births and deaths.
- It is best to phone and book a special appointment to save the family the distress of attending when other ceremonies may be going on.
- The family must present the death certificate to the registrar where the child died within 5 days of the child's death.
- The registrar will then issue the 'certificate for disposal'. This will allow the funeral directors to proceed with the funeral arrangements.

## Issuing a death certificate

- Best practice is that the doctor completing the death certificate should have seen the child in the last 14 days of life. If this has not been practical, the doctor can usually still issue a certificate following discussion with the coroner
- Verification and certification of death are not the same (see this section)

# Cremation

Cremation is becoming increasingly popular in the UK (70% of all registered deaths in 2001). Many religions have differing rules regarding cremation (see Chapter 20) and in some faiths this can also be dependent on the age of the child.

Certain legal rules have to be followed to allow cremation.

- The family must apply for cremation with Form 1.
- Then the doctor who completed the death certificate must complete Form 4.

    1 The doctor must see the body after death.
    2 He or she should have looked after the child for more than 24 hours.
    3 He or she should have seen the child within 14 days.

- If points 2 and 3 cannot be met then the doctor must discuss the case with the coroner and obtain permission that 'no further action is required'.
- The doctor who completed Form 4 must then bring in another medical practitioner who has neither attended nor been otherwise concerned with the care or treatment of the child and who is not a relative or partner of the medical practitioner signing Form 4.
- The second doctor then must examine the child's body and complete Form 5. He must also speak to either another doctor, nurse, or member of the family to ensure that they have no concerns regarding the cause of death. The family should be pre-warned about this as then may find it distressing to have an unknown doctor asking them questions and examining their child. Many religions also have rules about who can touch the child after death.
- Finally the 'authority to cremate' (Form 10) is signed by the medical referee for the crematorium.
- If the coroner has issued the death certificate, then Forms 4 and 5 are not required.

# Transporting the body

Irrespective of legal niceties, most police forces feel they have an obligation to treat with suspicion the discovery of any dead child in an unusual context. For this reason, funeral directors should always be the ones to transport a child's body.

Although some families may wish to transport the body home or to the hospice by car, this should be discouraged. Firstly, the driver may be emotionally upset and unsafe to drive the car. Secondly, if there is a crash and the police find a dead child in the car it is likely to cause serious legal problems. If this is very important to a family, the local police should be involved in the discussions from the outset.

# Organ donation

- Organ donation (subject to religious constraint) can be discussed with families who request it.
- Organ donation can give the family a sense of positivity and the feeling that something good might come out of their personal tragedy.
- Organs can only be donated if they are healthy. Unfortunately, due to the nature of many of the paediatric deaths seen in life-limited disorders, actual donation from this group is low.
- Cases where organ donation is not allowed include:
  - malignancy (except primary brain tumours);
  - genetic and neurodegenerative disorders affecting multiple organs;
  - HIV;
  - viral hepatitis;
  - major sepsis.
- Most organ donations come from trauma cases via paediatric intensive care units.

# Post mortem

Post mortem may be requested for a number of reasons:
- looking at the effects of the illness on specific parts of the body;
- getting biopsies from tissue that would not otherwise be available, e.g. brain tissue;
- trying to obtain information to confirm diagnosis.

In all these situations (subject to religious constraint) parents may well give permission for a post mortem. This is particularly so if they feel it may help other children with similar conditions or when a genetic diagnosis may have an influence on future pregnancies.

It is important to remember that parents will see 'tissue' or 'pathology' samples or 'organs' differently from the medical view. To them, these are parts of their child. This is particularly true of some organs such as heart and brain.

- It is always important to reassure the parents that:
  - the procedure is surgical and the child would be sutured up afterwards;
  - all organs and tissue would be replaced unless specific consent is given to retain certain tissues or organs;
  - dependent on the circumstances post mortem can be limited to certain areas, tissues, or organs;
  - the child's face would not be damaged;
  - the child's body would be respected throughout the process;
  - the doctors will arrange to talk to the parents afterwards about any of the findings if the parents so wish.

# Looking after the body

## In the home

- Under normal circumstances a child's body can be kept in the home for up to 2–3 days.
- In warmer weather this time frame is reduced.
- It would be prudent to put a waterproof cover on the child's bed.
- Cotton wool can be put as a plug into the anus.
- It is important that any room used in the family's house has free flow of air.
- Home air conditioning units can be used.
- Air fresheners can be helpful.
- It is important to keep all insects out of the room.
- For longer periods of time the funeral directors can take the child's body to their offices and embalm it, and then return it back within several hours.

## At the hospice

- Most children's hospices have 'special rooms'.
- These look like and are the size of normal bedrooms but have an industrial level refrigeration unit attached to allow the room to cool down.
- The child's body can be kept longer without the need for embalming.
- Parents can grieve whilst having the benefits of the internal bereavement support structures and resources of the hospice.
- The parents can access the child's body at any time. Parents often wish to see the child in the evening or at night.
- The bereavement support team can help:
  - the families adjust to the loss of the child;
  - if required with washing, dressing, putting the child into the coffin;
  - to collect items for a memory box;
  - the siblings if they wish to see the child's body;
  - with follow up support for the whole family for whatever length of time is required.
- The child can be taken straight from the 'special room' to the funeral.

## At the hospital

- The child's body can be stored in the hospital mortuary.
- All hospitals have a chapel of rest where family and friends can view the body.

## At the funeral director's

- The child's body can be stored in the funeral director's mortuary.
- All funeral directors have a chapel of rest where family and friends can view the body.
- The funeral director's offices are often near the family's home.

# Coroner

The coroner is either a lawyer or doctor (often both) who is responsible for investigating unnatural or sudden deaths of which the cause is unknown.

The coroner's authority is conducted through the police force. This is important as families, unless pre-warned, may become distressed at seeing police cars outside their house or police officers inside their homes.

The coroner needs to be informed in all of the following cases.

- where the deceased was not attended during his last illness by a registered medical practitioner;
- if the registrar has been unable to obtain a duly completed certificate of cause of death, or where it appears to the registrar from the particulars contained in such certificate, or otherwise, that the deceased was not seen by the certifying medical practitioner *either* after death *or* within 14 days;
- where the cause of death appears to be unknown;
- if the registrar has reason to believe that the death was unnatural or caused by violence or neglect, or by abortion, or was attended by suspicious circumstance;
- where it appears to the registrar that the death occurred during an operation or before recovery from the effects of an anaesthetic: *or*
- it appears to the registrar from the contents of any medical certificate that the death was due to industrial disease or industrial poisoning;
- if the deceased had an operation in the preceding 6 months that might be related to cause of death.

If a doctor suspects any of the above, then the following needs to occur.
- The doctor calls the coroner's office.
- The doctor should inform the parents.
- The family cannot refuse to have the coroner involved.
- Nothing should be touched around the child; the body should not be moved.
- No tubes, lines, or instruments can be removed without prior discussion with the coroner.
- The coroner's officers will take details from all the health care professionals and the family.
- The coroner's officers will arrange for the child's body to be transferred by funeral directors to an approved hospital for post mortem.

Subsequently the coroner will obtain information from all the sources. He or she has three options.
1 If the child's doctor can provide a legal death certificate then the coroner can approve the certificate to the registrar.
2 If the child's doctor cannot provide a legal death certificate, then the coroner can authorize a post mortem (the family cannot refuse this). From the post mortem the coroner can issue a death certificate.
3 If the death falls into certain categories then the coroner can call an inquest with or without jury.

# References

**1** Smale, D.A. (2002). *Law of burial, cremation and exhumation*, 7th edn. Shaw and Sons, Crayford, Kent.

**2** Brook, L. and Hain, R. (2008). Predicting death in children. *Arch. Dis. Child.* **93** (12), 1067–70.

# Religion and ritual

# Introduction

Religion and ritual have featured in human society for many thousands of years. The fact that they have survived and are still embraced by cultures across the world exemplifies their use and the benefits to human kind. Over time many rituals have changed and been modified as society develops and integrates, with migration playing its part. This can lead to different rituals within different cultures of the same religion. When this happens the danger of stereotyping should always be borne in mind.

The complexity of the rituals of different religions and their diversity can seem overwhelming at times but, interestingly, all religions appear to follow many similar themes, particularly surrounding death. Even though each culture has its own approach to death, in almost all faiths death is seen as a time of transition.

The rituals surrounding death can allow a release of emotions with support from the community around the bereaved. Pathological grief is sometimes seen when this support is not available, particularly for immigrants who do not have local cultural links.

Many individual factors such as age, gender, and cause of death of the child can influence how the family responds in terms of the rituals they adopt. Even if these may appear to contrast strongly with our own beliefs it is important to respect the family's wishes and support them appropriately. This view should also encompass respecting their individual ritual specialist.

With the changes occurring within society it is important to recognize that different generations may behave differently in response to death within the same culture. Also, people are not necessarily familiar with their own religious ritual around death.

Finally, we need to recognize that even individuals who say they do not belong to a particular religion or faith may hold very strong ethical and spiritual beliefs. It is equally important to understand these beliefs and support the individual appropriately.

# Christianity

- Christians believe that there is only one God and that Jesus Christ is the 'Son of God' who was sent to save mankind.
- Their religious beliefs stem from events recorded in the Bible.
- They believe that those who repent of their sins and turn to Jesus Christ will be forgiven and will join him in heaven after death.
- Over time many subgroups have appeared, but the largest group worldwide is represented by Catholics. There is such great variation in traditions that it is important to check with each family regarding their individual denomination.

## Symbols and spiritual advisers
- The symbol is the cross of Christ.
- Spiritual advisors vary depending on the particular denomination or sect. They range from priests or vicars to religious elders.

## Specific issues
- Some faiths may fast for Lent.
- There are normally no objections to organ donations.
- There are many sects with individual laws, such as the restriction of Jehovah's Witnesses regarding blood transfusion.

## Before and after death for Catholics (variations for other denominations)
- A priest can be called to anoint the dying child and provide spiritual support to the child and family.
- Privacy should be provided.
- Babies can be baptized.
- Mass is part of the funeral service.
- Non-Catholics cannot take communion.

**Visiting the home or church** There are no special limitations or rules beyond common courtesies.

## Funeral
- The body can be buried or cremated.
- The open coffin can be displayed in the church on the night before the burial and a vigil kept.
- The common structure of the funeral service is
  - the bidding;
  - the word;
  - prayer;
  - the commendation;
  - the committal.

Many other Christian groups have simpler versions of this.

**Anniversary of death** There are no special rules but many families find it helpful to attend a remembrance service or follow a specific ritual on special dates or anniversaries.

# Islam

- Islam is one of the most commonly held religions worldwide, and the second largest in the UK.
- Muslims believe that there is only one God (Allah) and that Muhammad (peace be on him) was the last of a line of prophets.
- The holy book is called the Qur'an.
- Muslims believe in life after death in the form of resurrection at the day of judgement. Death is predetermined by God and death and suffering are part of God's plan.
- There are five pillars to the faith:
  - belief in one God;
  - daily prayers;
  - fasting during Ramadan;
  - giving alms (2.5% of income);
  - pilgrimage to Makkah (Hajj).

## Symbols and spiritual advisers

- Symbols are the crescent moon and star.
- Islam has no ordained priesthood. Each community has its own local spiritual leader, the 'Imam', who performs religious duties including teaching.

## Specific issues

- The extended family is important and decisions often require the approval of the head of the family (not always the father of the child).
- Young children are not expected to fast during Ramadan. From the age of 7 years the children may fast for a few specific days with their parents. From the age of 12 years they will often fast for the full month.
- Any adult or child who is ill can be excused from fasting.
- Muslims believe in life after death, and as such it is important to continue in a form that makes the preservation of the body essential. Thus, they do not agree with organ donation and accept post mortem examinations only if legally required.
- Pork and pork products are prohibited, as is the meat of other animals that is not 'halal' (killed according to Islamic law).

## Before and after death

- Before death, family members may sit with the child and read verses from the Qur'an.
- The child should face Makkah.
- The Declaration of faith (Shahada) is said.
- Holy water may be placed in the child's mouth.
- Just before death a family member may whisper into the child's ear the call to prayer.
- After death:
  - the child is laid flat;
  - their face is pointed towards Makkah;
  - their feet are put together;
  - their arms to the side;
  - their eyes closed;

- their chin is wrapped in cloth to prevent mouth opening;
- their body is washed by same-sex members of the family;
- their body is shrouded in white linen without any religious emblems.
- The body should not be touched by non-Muslims.
- Do not remove any religious objects or threads.
- Children are not permitted to attend rituals. They are discouraged from asking questions and are expected to forget death as soon as possible.

## Visiting the home or mosque

- There is a very strict social etiquette within the community.
  - Men and women normally worship separately: men at the mosque and women at home.
  - Men and women do not normally shake hands.
  - Women should dress modestly.
- If visiting the mosque, there may be separate entrances for men and women. Men cover their heads and women are expected to cover their heads, arms, and legs.
- Muslim families adopt an open house to those people paying their respects after a child's death.
  - Shoes should be removed when entering the home.
  - Red should not be worn.

## Funeral

- The child should be buried within 24 hours by men.
- The grave is aligned so that the child's face can be turned sideways to face Makkah.
- Women and children do not attend the burial but can attend the funeral ceremony at the mosque.
- Flowers are normally accepted.
- After burial prayers are said at the mosque or home and then the family will eat.
- There is great variation in expression of grief. Some sects lament loudly; others maintain serene stoicism.
- On the 3rd, 7th, and 40th day after the death the men will gather to say prayers.
- Mourning normally lasts 3 days with the family staying indoors; then for up to 40 days the grave can be visited and alms given to the poor.

## Anniversary of death
On the first anniversary a ceremony is held, prayers are said, and food served. A stone may be placed on the grave.

# Hinduism

- Hinduism is the oldest religion in the world and the third largest in the UK.
- Hindus believe in a Supreme Spirit that represents an Ultimate Reality.
- Because it is not possible for humans to comprehend this Supreme Spirit, they worship the different aspects of the universe in which it resides. These aspects are personalized as gods and deity.
- The 3 key gods are:
  - Brahma the Creator;
  - Vishnu the Preserver;
  - Shiva the Destroyer.
- Hindus believe in reincarnation based on the actions in one's life (karma).

## Symbols and spiritual advisers

- The symbol Om is regarded as sacred.
- Hindus have many sacred texts. The oldest are the Vedas.
- The Bhagavad-Gita is the most widely read.
- Hindu priests (pandits) perform holy rites.

## Specific issues

- Hindus have very strong extended family ties.
- Families often have small shrines within the home.
- There are no religious objections to organ donation or post mortem examination.
- Many Hindus are vegetarian and almost all do not eat beef. The right hand is used for eating and the left hand is used for personal hygiene.

## Before and after death

- Before death family members may sit with the child and read prayers.
- Holy water from the Ganges and the sacred Tulsi leaf may be placed in the child's mouth.
- A child should die whilst hearing the name of God.
- At the time of death the family may grieve loudly.
- After death:
  - the child is laid flat sometimes lifted to the floor;
  - the body is washed by the family;
  - the body is wrapped in a white shroud or white clothes;
  - the body is placed in a coffin and a coin, gold piece, or Tulsi leaf is placed in their mouth;
  - the face is left uncovered;
  - the body is anointed and garlanded with flowers.
- The body should be touched as little as possible.
- Do not remove any religious objects or threads.

## Visiting the home or temple

- Normal social courtesies apply.
- Shoes should be removed when entering the home.
- If entering a room with a shrine in the house, then shoes should be removed and women should cover their heads.

- In the temple everyone must remove shoes and women should cover their heads.
- People can pray individually or as a congregation.

## Funeral

- Hindus are cremated, although young babies may be buried.
- The child should be cremated within 24 hours.
- Flowers are accepted.
- The body is normally taken home first and then by the family to the temple before going to the crematorium.
- The mourners walk around the body in an anticlockwise direction to symbolize the unwinding of the thread of life.
- The ashes are scattered in running water.
- Mourning normally lasts for 10 days (but can last up to 40 days) during which time the family wear white.
- On the 11th or 13th day a final ceremony is held.
- Money is given to charity.

## Anniversary of death

- On anniversaries a ceremony is held, prayers are said, and food served.
- The family may not attend other religious festivals in the first year.

# Sikhism

- Sikhism is one of the newest religions in the world and the fourth largest in the UK.
- Sikhs believe in one God.
- They believe in equality of all people and that life should involve work, worship, and charity.
- Sikhism rejects ritual.
- They believe in reincarnation and karma.
- The religion was founded in the 15th century by Guru Nanak.
- The Sikh holy book is the Guru Granth Sahib.

### Symbols and spiritual advisers

- The Sikh symbol is the khanda.
- There are 5 religious symbols (known as the '5 Ks') of great importance to Sikhs:
  1 kesh: uncut hair;
  2 kangha: comb;
  3 karra: ridged bangle worn on the right wrist;
  4 kacha: a pair of shorts;
  5 kirpaan: a short sword.
- Sikhs have no specific religious hierarchy but each temple has a group of elders.

### Specific issues

- There are no religious objections to organ donation or post mortem examinations.
- Many Sikhs are vegetarian and almost all those who eat meat will not eat beef. The right hand is used for eating and the left for personal hygiene.

### Before and after death

- Before death family members may sit with the child and read prayers.
- Holy water or Amrit may be placed in the child's mouth.
- A child should die whilst hearing the name of God, Waheguru (wonderful Lord), being recited.
- Generally Sikhs are happy for non-Sikhs to tend the body.
- After death:
  - the body is washed and dressed by the same sex members of the family;
  - the body is covered in a white sheet;
  - many parents would wish for their child to wear the 5 Ks and an older child a turban;
  - the body is placed in a coffin and gifts of dried fruit, clothes, or money may be put in.
- Do not remove any religious objects or threads.

### Visiting the home or temple (Gurudwara)

- Normal social courtesies apply.
- Shoes should be removed when entering the home.

- In the temple everyone must remove shoes and both men and women should cover their heads.
- On entering the prayer room all worshippers bow their heads in front of the Guru Granth Sahib.

## Funeral

- Sikhs are cremated, although young babies may be buried.
- The child should be cremated within 24 hours.
- Flowers are accepted.
- The body is normally taken home first and then to the Gurudwara before going to the crematorium.
- The ashes are scattered in running water.
- Mourning normally lasts for 10 days during which time the family wear white.
- During this time there is normally a complete reading of the Guru Granth Sahib.
- Money is given to charity.

**Anniversary of death** There are no special rules, but many families find it helpful to attend a remembrance service or follow a specific ritual on special dates or anniversaries.

# Judaism

- Judaism is one of the oldest monotheistic religions of the world.
- Jews believe in one God with whom they have a covenant.
- Judaism has many texts but the main one is the Torah.
- Orthodox Jews follow the traditional interpretation of the will of God in the Torah.
- Progressive Jews follow a modern interpretation of the ancient laws.
- Two of the Jewish commandments are to honour the dead and comfort the mourners.

## Symbols and spiritual advisers

- The Jewish symbol is the Star of David.
- Spiritual leaders are known as Rabbis.

## Specific issues

- There are many variations in Jewish custom at time of death.
- Hasidic Jews do not shake hands with women and prefer not to look at or speak with them.
- Orthodox Jews require kosher food (with certain rituals attached).
- They also do not allow organ donation with the exception of cornea.
- All Jews decline post mortem examinations unless legally required.

### Before and after death

- Before death the rabbi should be called to recite specific prayers.
- At the point of death no one should leave the room.
- Generally only the family should handle the body; non-Jews should wear gloves.
- After death:
  - the body is tended by family of the same sex;
  - the body is covered in a sheet;
  - eyes are closed and mouth closed with the lower jaw bound;
  - the body is straightened with the feet pointing to the door;
  - a candle is lit and placed near the head;
  - mirrors are covered;
  - some orthodox Jews may lay the body on the floor for 20min and pour water outside the door;
  - others may put ashes on the eyes;
- From death until burial the body is guarded.
- Do not remove any religious objects or threads.

## Visiting the home or temple (synagogue)

- Normal social courtesies apply.
- Strict orthodox Jews may prefer not to have home visits on the Sabbath and prefer same sex doctors and nurses.
- In orthodox synagogues, men and women sit separately and both men and women cover their heads.

## Funeral

- Jews are buried although some liberal Jews will be cremated.
- The child should be buried within 24 hours.

- Flowers are not accepted.
- Funerals are simple and unostentatious.
- Gentiles may attend the funeral but not the internment.
- No mourning is carried out if a baby dies within 30 days of birth.
- The Shiva (7 days of mourning) starts after the burial:
  - 3 days of private weeping and mourning;
  - then 4 days of shared mourning with friends.
  - prayer of Kaddish said daily.
  - Gentiles are welcome.
- The Sheloshim (30 days) during which the family does not shave or cut their hair. Kaddish recited daily.
- For next 10 months the Kaddish recited weekly by the men.
- Money is given to charity.

## Anniversary of death

- On the 1st anniversary (Yahrzeit) the tombstone is unveiled. Visitors place a small stone on it.
- Yizkor is an annual Jewish holiday when the dead are thought of in a memorial service and candles are lit.

# Buddhism

- Buddhists do not worship a God or deities.
- Instead they strive for personal spiritual development to focus on the true meaning of life.
- Their teaching is based on non-violence and compassion for all forms of life.

## Symbols and spiritual advisers

- Buddhists may have many religious symbols but none that are mandatory.
- Spiritual leaders in the community as well as monks and nuns.

## Specific issues

- Buddhists believe in reincarnation.
- Their faith has a strong affinity with death and they accept death as a process of rebirth, leading to higher levels of enlightenment.
- Their philosophy encompasses the issue of impermanence of life with suffering and as such bearing suffering with dignity and equanimity.
- Organ donation and post mortem are permitted.

## Before and after death

- No special requirements.
- As death occurs local monks and members of the family's local society will say prayers and support the bereaved family.
- The body can be washed.
- It is wrapped in a sheet without emblems.

**Visiting the home or temple** Normal social courtesies apply.

## Funeral

- Cremation is the norm although burial is also permitted.
- There is great variation in the form of the funeral rites dependent on the Buddhist group.
- There is a calm acceptance of death.

**Anniversary of death** No formal procedure.

# Traditional African approaches to a child's death

There is no single 'African approach'. Cultural diversity between southern and northern tribes in Uganda is perhaps greater than between European Caucasians, Australian Aborigines, North American Inuit, and South Asian Indians. Furthermore, in modern Africa, traditional beliefs are often blended with 'Western' religion, so that traditional and Western beliefs regarding health and healing, illness and injury, and death and dying weave inextricably together around the death of children.

Some common beliefs that do span across the different cultures in sub Saharan Africa, however, have implications for children's palliative care in many diverse African countries and cultures.

Traditional African healing is very much focused on restoring wholeness and peace. 'God' is seen as the ultimate healer and curer and doctor, helped by his divine intermediaries and the good living–dead ancestors, the diviners, who can find the cause, the local doctors who can find the cure, and the caring and loving family and community who can make all the above possible. In particular it tries to restore wholeness and peace between the sick person and:

- God, the ancestors, and the living;
- the family;
- the community and its basic beliefs and values.

Some commonly held beliefs that influence children's palliative care include the following:

- The belief that life is a great gift and therefore its preservation and prolongation is the central duty of every person, family, and community, which can make it difficult for families to move from a curative to a palliative approach if health workers do not discover and gently challenge it.
- The belief that illness and death (especially in childhood) do not come randomly or independently. Rather, that some enemy (living or dead) must have caused it. This can continue to distract the child and family into searching for external agents and seeking redress rather than using the limited time left to them in a constructive, peaceful, and supportive way.
- The belief that 'blessings of all sorts come from fulfilling the duty to care for the terminally sick'. This belief sits fairly easily with children's palliative care as it provides a strong spiritual driver for the family to pull together to do as much as they can to care for the child.
- The belief that a 'good death':
  - comes in old age;
  - is not sudden;
  - allows the patient to make preparations, forgive, and reconcile with all;
  - allows the patient to be able to see their dear ones and bid them farewell.

- Death in childhood is rarely seen as a good death, and the family may need help to focus on all that has been good in a child's life, to feel that life has not been wasted, and to understand that children too have affairs that need to be put in order and farewells that need to be said.
- The belief in the importance of death rituals. Traditional African beliefs put great importance on correct rituals after the death of the child. The particular rituals vary, but there are common themes; particularly around:
  - burying the dead child close to (or within) the family home;
  - not tempting fate by bringing death of very young infants too close to the mother or surviving siblings in case further childbirth is prevented or surviving children themselves succumb.

In most cases these rituals seem to serve to complete the circle of life; appease ancestral spirits and allow the surviving family to move forward unencumbered by unfulfilled obligations from the past.

Ultimately, if a single 'African traditional approach' to healing can be articulated, it is the aim for a sick person to be completely at peace with themselves, to collect together their fears and overcome them, to be assured that their desires and wishes will be dealt with and that their anxieties and aspirations will be catered for by the ones they love. All these modes of healing are necessary for the children who are dying and their families. Together they form part of an integrated healing or holistic approach that is culturally appropriate.

## Essential reading

Murray Parkes, C., Laungani, P., and Young, B. (ed.) (2006). *Death and bereavement across cultures.* Routledge, London.

Goldman, A., Hain, R., and Liben, S. (ed.) (2006). *Oxford textbook of palliative care for children,* Chapters 14 and 16. Oxford University Press, Oxford.

## Acknowledgement

Special thanks to Dr Narinder Saund and the multifaith group Leicestershire and Dr Justin Amery for the section on traditional African approaches.

# Bereavement

# Introduction

It is said that there are only two certainties in life, 'death and taxes'. Death is very much part of the normal life cycle of all living creatures. Death generates different levels of grief in people, most often linked to our relationship with the individual and our social cultural upbringing. Up to 100 years ago in the Western world, death was commonplace and was seen by all age groups. However, in the present day Western world death is seen much less often and often perceived as a failure of medical technology and skills.

Society and individuals appear to accept the death of the elderly much more easily than the death of a child. The elderly are often seen as having had a good life and achieved many goals. Because our young remain immature and vulnerable for so many years, nature gives us a very powerful parent–child bond. The loss seen with the breaking of the bond generates intense emotion and grief.

As paediatric palliative care professionals dealing with the family, we are looked towards by other health care professionals and society to help deal with the bereavement and its associated grief. It is important to recognize that it is not our sole responsibility.

- Many cultures have strong religious rituals that are used to support and comfort the family. Many families will look towards their religious community and leaders for support.
- Other families will choose the support within their extended family.
- Finally, the community around a family can be very supportive.

What all these groups lack, because of the small numbers of child deaths, is an understanding of what to expect with the bereavement and how to help with the grief process.

# Bereavement theory

Over the last 90 years the theories around paediatric bereavement have slowly evolved from Freud to the 'stage models', up to our current theories of grief based around 'relearning'. It is helpful to understand the basis of some of these theories. In reality we use elements from all the theories to help the family.

## Stage model[1–4]

1 Immediately after death: disbelief and denial.
2 Protest phase with loud crying, motor restlessness, and agitation. Lasting a few weeks or months.
3 Mourning phase where the patient enters a depressive type phase. Lasting a few months up to the second anniversary of death.
4 Adaptation to the loss.

The weakness of this 'medical' model is that it oversimplifies the whole grief process for the parents and family. It compartmentalizes and sets time parameters for the whole process, with a definite end 'when all is well'. In reality, individuals in families grieve at different rates, in different ways, and often flip from one stage to another over time.

## Grief work model[5,6]

- Accepts that grieving takes time and that it is dependent on the individual.
- Grief requires a holistic approach to the individual's needs.
- The individual will need support with personal and emotional issues as well as help with their interaction with society.
- Gives guidance to caregivers in terms of actively challenging the loss by supporting the 'tasks' of grieving.

## Relationship with the child model[7,8]

As with the grief work model but with the additional perspectives:
- the grief process represents an ending of one relationship with the child, and forming a new relationship with the child;
- the new relationship is long term;
- the parents continue to remember the child;
- understanding the unique suffering that individuals go through.

# Bereavement issues for children

The chronically ill child with a life-limiting condition may well experience many personal bereavement issues before their death.

- There is the loss of their normal childhood.
- Loss of the physical ability to do things other children do.
- Loss of the ability to develop normal relationships with school friends and members of the opposite sex.
- Sadness at seeing how hard their parents and families have to struggle to look after them.
- Losses suffered as they see their own health deteriorate knowing this represents further loss of function of their body with the threat of death approaching.
- Children with similar medical conditions experience grief as they see their friends with life-limiting conditions dying around them.

Discussion about death with the child not only helps the child cope with the future but can also significantly help parents with their bereavement and grief.[9]

# Bereavement issues for siblings

Siblings often experience behavioural problems.

- The normal behaviour of siblings is linked to rivalry for parental attention. When their brother or sister has a life-limiting condition this norm is broken, as the parents concentrate all their attentions on the ill child.
- A large number of siblings develop behavioural problems as a result of bereavement. Research in this group of children is limited. However the issues that appear to affect their reaction are both general and also developmentally specific.
- Young children tend to be egocentric so they can sometimes feel that their negative thoughts towards their sibling either caused or exacerbated the sibling's illness.
- Because deaths are rare and children are normally 'protected' by adults they have limited experience of what a dead person looks like, or what their reaction to death should be.
- Children of all ages have vivid imaginations. If no attempt is made to explain, in terms they understand, what is happening to their sibling, then they will start to make up their own ideas from the limited information they hear and based on their limited life experience. As in life, what is imagined is often worse than reality.

# Bereavement issues for parents

The way a parent may grieve is dependent on a number of issues.

- The parents' premorbid personality and psychiatric history. Parents with previous anxiety or depression have been shown to be at greater risk of abnormal grief reactions.
- Whether the death was sudden and unexpected, or foreseeable after a prolonged illness. The former parents have intense issues with disbelief, denial, and seeking behaviour. The latter group of parents often experience long periods of grief as they see their child slowly deteriorating.
- Many parents have to combine grief with guilt, particularly when the child may have had a genetic disorder.
- Others find they that they need to direct their anger phase at someone—God, their health care professionals, or spouse.
- Many marriages come under strain and fail as the couple struggle to remodel their relationship without the child.
- During the illness of a child many parents lose their normal social circle of friends and family. They replace this with a circle of health care professionals to whom they become very attached. These same parents feel rejected after the death of a child as they find the health care professionals leave to concentrate on the next family. The same happens to social/financial benefits, as they are lost after the child dies and this can lead to significant financial hardship.
- Religion and ritual can have a great effect on parents' grief reactions (see Chapter 20). Many benefit greatly from their faiths and the rituals of shared grief with family and friends, particularly around the funeral. Others can find the process distressing if it is imposed on them by the society around them, and they have to participate in things they do not agree with.
- Parents who have a number of children with life-limiting conditions may struggle greatly with grief. They may have already gone through the grief of losing another child. They may have to cope with looking after a sibling knowing that they will have to go through the same grief again in the future.
- In the past it was felt that, with time, parents would get over the death of their child. Now the thinking is more to do with the parents coming to terms with the death of the child. However, the timescale of this process is uncertain. It was thought in the past to take 1 year, and abnormal grief was diagnosed if it continued for over 2 years. The newer models of grief work and personal experience suggests that rigid time framing is inappropriate. The process of developing a new relationship with the dead child for parents may take years[10] and abnormal grief should be considered if the parent fails to make progress in the tasks of grieving.

# Bereavement issues for society

The death of a child has a profound effect on the community around the child. A great many people are emotionally affected and it is important to reflect on some of these groups.

**Grandparents** The grief felt by grandparents is twofold. Not only do they have to deal with the death of their grandchild but they also have to deal with the sadness of seeing their own children grieving.

**Schools** The death of a child can be a source of great distress to their school friends. For children this may be their first contact with death. For school teachers there is the difficulty of knowing how to handle the situation.

# Managing bereavement

There is a common misconception that child bereavement support needs to come from specialists and counsellors. In reality this is just not true. Parents obtain most of the support and help through grief from family, friends, and society.[10] Work has shown that normal psychological models of counselling may not be effective.[11,12] However, early support from bereavement support teams can help parents greatly in their grief process.[10] These multidisciplinary teams can help by:

• listening in a non-judgemental way;
• acting as sounding boards for parents, as they try various approaches in the journey through their grief;
• helping parents to maintain a link with the child through memory boxes, etc.;
• helping parents to look at the grief process as journey of steps and not something that has to tackled all in one go;
• supporting parents when things are going badly;
• helping parents through the various emotions of anger, guilt, sadness, and loss;
• helping guide parents as they endeavour to develop new relationships and new ways of working;
• supporting siblings by communication through talking, group work, art therapy, and music therapy—all of these techniques can be used with siblings before, at the time, and after the death of a child;
• recognizing and embracing the silent suffering seen in grandparents and supporting them through their grief;
• giving advice to schools as to how to approach the issues around death in the school assembly and classroom;
• identifying when grief enters an abnormal phase and initiating specialist medical intervention.

## References

**1** Bowlby, J. and Parkes, C.M. (1970). Separation and loss within the family. In *The child in his family* (ed. E.J. Anthony and C. Koupernik), pp. 197–216. Wiley: New York.

**2** Engel, G.L. (1964). Grief and grieving. *Am. J. Nurs.* **64**, 93–8.

**3** Osterweis, M., Solomon, F., and Green, M. (1984). *Bereavement: reactions, consequences and care.* National Academy Press, Washington DC.

**4** Rosenblatt, P.C., Walsh, R.P., and Jackson, D.A. (1976). *Grief and mourning in cross cultural perspective.* HRAF Press, New Haven, Connecticut.

**5** Parkes, C.M. and Weiss, R. (1983). *Recovery from bereavement.* Basic Books, New York.

**6** Worden, W. (1991). *Grief counselling and grief therapy: a handbook for the mental health practitioner*, 2nd edn. Springer Publishing Co, New York.

**7** Attig, T.W. (1996). *We grieve: relearning the world.* Oxford University Press, New York.

**8** Davies, B., Attig, T.W., and Towne, M. (2006). Bereavement. In *Oxford textbook of palliative care for children* (ed. A. Goldman, R. Hain, and S. Liben), pp. 193–203. Oxford University Press, Oxford.

**9** Kreicbergs, U., Valdimarsdottir, U., Henter, J.-I., and Steineck, G. (2004). Talking about death with children who have severe malignant disease. *N. Engl. J. Med.* **351** (12), 1175–86.

**10** Kreicbergs, U., Lannen, P., Onelov, E., and Wolfe, J. (2007). Parental grief after losing a child to cancer: impact of professional and social support on long-term outcomes. *J. Clin. Oncol.* **25** (22), 3307–12.

**11** Jordan, J.R. and Neimeyer, R.A. (2003). Does grief counselling work? *Death Studies* **27** (9), 765–86.

**12** Stroebe, W., Schut, H., and Stroebe, M.S. (2005). Grief work, disclosure and counseling: do they help the bereaved? *Clin. Psychol. Rev.* **25** (4), 395–414.

# Communication skills

# Introduction

The medical care of children is characterized by the extent to which it relies on collaboration with family. In effect, the family of a child is expected to behave as colleagues with the paediatric or primary care team. It is expected that they will:
- always be available to the child;
- have the child's best interests at heart;
- be able to work alongside medical and nursing staff.

The goal of communication with patients and families is to ensure the families feel confident and competent in this collegiate relationship (see box).

Factors that can complicate this include:
- prior understandings and misunderstandings;
- emotional coping mechanisms (e.g. denial);
- discordance between the way information is given and received (e.g. differences in vocabulary between professional and family);
- difficulty in remembering information.

The aim of communication is twofold:
1  to exchange information between family and professional;
2  to minimize the inherent imbalance of power between professional and lay person in a hospital setting.

The aim of what follows is to provide a structure that also illustrates some of the important principles of information giving and empathy.

The goal of good communication is to enable the family of a child or young person to become competent colleagues in his or her medical care through the following:
- Imparting factual information and understanding:
  - to an appropriate level
  - at an appropriate pace
  - using appropriate language.
- Imparting a sense of participation in the team through:
  - seeking the family's perspective
  - empathic acknowledgement (implied and overt) of their concerns
  - soliciting the views of child and/or family in decision making.

# Setting the scene

- Families find discussions with doctors intimidating and need positive encouragement to volunteer information.
- The aim of setting the scene is to provide a physical and temporal space to facilitate this.
- This usually takes planning. Impromptu communication should be avoided if possible. It is better to arrange a discussion at a specific time and place.

### Physical space

- Privacy. Where possible a separate room with the door closed. If necessary, at least draw curtains around the bed.
- A quiet room.
- Comfortable furnishings that allow professional and family to be on the same physical level.

### Temporal space

- Set aside time, ideally by arranging an appointment (and keeping to it).
- Unhurried atmosphere, e.g. by sitting down rather than standing, avoiding talking too fast.
- Minimize interruption, e.g. switch off bleeps and mobile phones.
- Avoid consulting a watch.

### Remove barriers

- No desk separating doctor from family.
- Eye contact on the same level, emphasizing equality.
- Maintaining eye contact is often interpreted to mean that professionals are not being entirely truthful.

### Have the facts straight

- Make sure you feel knowledgeable enough on the subject. If necessary, ask a senior colleague to be present or to facilitate the discussion.
- Do not delegate this important task to inappropriate members of the team (e.g. very junior medical or nursing colleagues).
- Recognize the importance that families give to discussions with doctors.
- Communicate results accurately. If not certain, admit it rather than risk giving inaccurate information.

### Who else should be there?

- Both parents if possible.
- 'Significant others', e.g. grandparents.
- A member of the nursing staff.
- Consider including the child or young person themselves if you are comfortable.

# Alignment

## Purpose of alignment

The aim is to understand what things look like from the family's perspective, by establishing what they already know, perceive, and understand.

▶ *This means they need to be able to talk first* and to explain:

- what they have already been told;
- their understanding of what they have been told;
- any relevant prior experience and its impact (e.g. the parents of a child newly diagnosed with leukaemia may have had experience of adult cancer that will inform—often erroneously—their understanding of it;
- what vocabulary they use. Insistence on an accurate technical term in preference to the family's own preferred term (e.g. 'tumour' rather than 'cancer') risks riding roughshod over important understanding and coping mechanisms and will compromise the effectiveness of communication.

## Tools to assist alignment

*Open questions* allow the family to set the agenda of the discussion, allowing free rein in interpretation of the question. Open questions can provide rich and varied information, but can jeopardize good communication if they become too unfocused or removed from the point.

*Closed questions* are used to obtain specific items of information, such as 'has anyone in your family had this condition before?' Overuse of closed questions can restrict discussions and prevent important issues being addressed. Discussions with no closed questions can be poorly focused and unsatisfactory.

*Summarizing and checking* It is important to check that your interpretation of what you are being told is accurate. Summarizing and checking allows this, conveys that the physician has listened to what has been said, as well as offering families the opportunity to correct or confirm what has been understood.

# Imparting information

A collegiate relationship with families requires them to understand the information you give accurately, and to trust that it is truthful. This requires:
- an appropriate level of information;
- given at an appropriate pace.

## Appropriate level of information

Information should:
- be enough to make any necessary decisions in an informed way;
- be enough to allay unnecessary fears;
- be enough to understand the significance of the results of tests that have been done and are immediately planned;
- not overwhelm and obscure what is really important;
- be given using appropriate terminology (avoiding jargon, use family's own terms where possible);
- be relevant. Avoid discussions about increasingly remote possibilities.

▶ The need for information correlates only poorly with perceived educational level. Prior assumptions about a family's intellectual ability risk being patronizing to some and incomprehensibly technical to others.

## Appropriate pace

The pace at which information is given should:
- be tailored to the needs of the individual child and family;
- be regulated during the discussion as new needs become clear;
- be punctuated by summaries, reviews, and a chance to ask questions;
- be supported by written materials (printed or electronic) that can be accessed by families at their own rate.

# Checking

Once information has been imparted ask the family if:
- they have had enough information;
- their concerns have been addressed;
- they have any further questions.

Reassure families that:
- they are not expected to remember everything first time;
- the team is happy to be asked questions again;
- if the consultant is not there, other members of the team such as nurses on the ward are able to answer questions.

Be prepared to go over some things again if checking reveals they have not been understood well.

# Future plans

Discussions are important to families. Many will feel anxious that the discussion has ended and need to know that there will be future conversations.

- Introduce other members of the team.
- Refer to them during the conversation so that families recognize that yours is not the only expert voice.
- Ditto the primary care team if the child is to be discharged home.
- Make a further appointment to meet the family at a certain date or time.
- Be honest if there is the possibility that you will be late.
- Ensure that your plans for meeting again are acceptable to the family, particularly if the child is to be discharged.

## Summary

- Discussion of bad news begins with a process of finding out how the situation is seen by the patient and family
- This is followed by a period when the doctor gives information at a pace, level, and amount that the family can assimilate accurately and easily
- Check for understanding at intervals throughout the discussion and on completion
- Repeat information if necessary
- Make future plans, including arrangements for any follow up meeting

## Chapter 23

# Communication among professionals

# Introduction

Communication skills among professionals all centre on the basic ideology of team working. Team working has repeatedly been shown in both business and health to be effective. The World Health Organization affirms that primary health should involve all related sectors working together, including education and social services, in addition to health care, and that efforts should be made to coordinate these sectors.[1]

## General points

- Team working can only work effectively when the child and family are seen as central to the 'team', with all the professionals acting as spokes to the central hub of family (Fig. 23.1).
- On average, a disabled child has contact with 10 different professionals and attends 20 clinic visits a year.[2]
- All the children who require palliative care will have different requirements, but in common they need everyone to work together and be clear on their roles and responsibilities, to ensure that the child and family's needs are met in a supportive and timely manner.

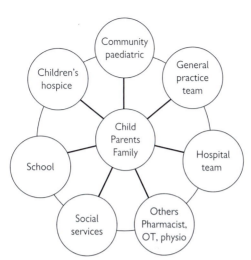

**Fig. 23.1** Professional involvement in the care of a child.

# Definitions

Team working can be defined as 'a group of individuals who share goals and work together to deliver services for which they are mutually accountable'.[3]

A variety of terms are used relating to the structure and philosophy of the teams; these include multidisciplinary, interdisciplinary, and transdisciplinary. These terms are not interchangeable but instead represent different forms of communication within teams.

### Multidisciplinary team working

In multidisciplinary team working, professionals collaborate and cooperate, but within their own set roles.
- Various professional groups meet together.
- Those with varying knowledge and skill bases meet together within a single agency.
- Different agencies meet together.

### Interdisciplinary team working

In interdisciplinary team working there is adaptation of roles, responsibilities, etc. to adjust to those of others in the team. This allows for integration of theoretical models and techniques.
- Professionals adapt their identified roles to interact with and take account of others in the group.
- There are adjustments to knowledge and skill bases.
- This results in various agency responsibilities.

### Transdisciplinary team working

In transdisciplinary team working there is a reformation of roles, knowledge, and skills to create family-centred cohesive services, with only one assessment.

# Team theory

A number of authors have written about how a team forms (Table 23.1). The pattern that emerges from all these models is that a team develops over time as individuals learn about each other's skill and knowledge. Roles are defined and responsibility is delegated. Conflict appears to be a natural event in the evolution of the team.

Handy[7] identified the factors required to develop a successful team (Table 23.2).

**Table 23.1** Models for the development of teams

| Lowe[8] | Roelofsen et al.[9] | Handy[7] |
|---|---|---|
| Becoming acquainted | Process-oriented | Forming |
| Trial and error | Result-oriented | Storming |
| Collective indecision | Problem-oriented | Norming |
| Crisis | Interdisciplinary team | Performing |
| Resolution | | |

**Table 23.2** Factors for a successful team

| **The givens** | |
|---|---|
| The group | Size, member characteristics, individual objectives, & stage of development |
| The task | Nature of the task; criteria of effectiveness, salience of task, & clarity of task |
| The environment | Norms and expectations, the leader position, intergroup relations, & the physical location |
| Intervening factors | Leadership style |
| | Process and procedure |
| | Motivation |
| Outcomes | Productivity |
| | Member satisfaction |

# Challenges of team working

There are considerable challenges involved in team working, particularly when one also looks at joint working at broader levels, including strategic planning and service commissioning.

## Organizational challenges

- Many organizations have their own way of working, hierarchy, pay, funding, geography, and training.
- Organizations have different ideologies, cultures, and attitudes.
- Organizational rigidity.
- Different levels of commitment.
- Time factors.
- Differing perceptions of the value of liaison.
- Attitude to leadership.
- Lack of training in team working or leadership skills.
- Power struggles over control and funding.
- Issues over justice of allocation of limited resources.
- Issues about individuals and the organizational value of their status or importance.
- Conflict can occur when either party does not complete their expected role and responsibilities, or blocks completion of goals set by others.
- Lack of understanding of the skills and roles of each other's profession.

## Communication problems

- Communication problems within each agency and also between them.
- Lack of understanding of need to communicate with particular groups, in particular, teachers, schools, and education.
- Use of language by professionals, particularly use of complex medical terms.
- Different interpretation of common language by different professionals, e.g. 'patient-centred', 'collaboration', or 'advocacy'.
- The complexity and rarity of the types of medical conditions means that knowledge of the conditions is restricted to a limited number of tertiary care specialist experts.

## 'Too many cooks'

Large numbers of professionals can be involved in looking after an individual child and family, particularly within the first year of diagnosis. The repeated contact by all these workers puts a major strain on family and child in terms of coordination, communication, understanding roles, developing relationships, and assessing which services are available. Parents will often complain that they feel swamped and suffocated by the number of people from the 'caring professions' they have to meet. The number of people involved can lead to inertia and confusion over care and responsibilities.

# Successful team working

Just as there are many challenges, so with some effort we can establish good effective team working.
- Planning ahead.
- Appropriate design and membership of the team.
- Allocation of time and funds.
- Appropriate location, facilities, and resources for the team.
- Good leadership based on skill rather than perceived status.
- Ability to change leadership as the needs of the child and family change.
- Leader able to coordinate individuals and organizations.
- Members to understand their own role and that of other members of the group.
- Respect for each other's knowledge and experience.
- Focused allocation of responsibilities and workload.
- Flexibility and compromise.
- Aim to set clear goals that are appropriate, specific, and measurable.
- Information to be disseminated in a clear understandable form to all members of the team, child, and family.

## Key worker

The identification of an appropriate person to act as key worker and as a coordinator is one suggestion to achieve effective teamwork to meet the palliative care needs of a child and family.

Some specific roles of a key worker have been identified, which include:
- information provision;
- identifying and addressing the child and family's needs;
- coordinating timely services;
- emotional support;
- acting in the role of advocate.

As with all services, the balance of these roles is dependent on the individual needs of the family and child. The key worker in effect takes on the role of 'team leader' for that child and family.

## References

**1** World Health Organization (1978). *Declaration of Alma-Ata*. WHO, New York.

**2** Sloper, P. (2002). *National service framework for children, External working group on Disabled Children—background work on key workers*. Department of Health, London. Available at ✆ www. doh.gov.uk/nsf/children/externalwgdisabled.htm

**4** Watson, D., Townsley, R., Abbott, D., and Latham, P. (2002). *Working together? Multi-agency working in services to disabled children with complex health care needs and their families. A literature review*. Handsel Trust Publications, Birmingham.

**5** Watson, D., Townsley, R., and Abbot, D. (2002). Exploring multi-agency working in services to disabled children with complex healthcare needs and their families. *J. Clin. Nurs.* **11**, 365–75.

**6** Pardess, E., Finzi, R., and Sever, J. (1993). Evaluating the best interests of the child—a model of multidisciplinary teamwork. *Med. Law* **12** (3–5), 205–11.

**7** Handy, C. (1993). *Understanding organizations*, 4th edn, pp. 150–79. Penguin, London.

**8** Lowe, J. and Herranen, M. (1978). Conflict in teamworking. *Social Work in Health Care* **3** (3), 323–30.

**9** Roelofsen, E.E., The, B.A., Beckerman, H., Lankhorst, G.J., and Bouter, L.M. (2002). Development and implementation of the Rehabilitation Activities Profile for children: impact on the rehabilitation team. *Clin. Rehabil.* **16** (4), 441–53.

# Coping skills

# Introduction

Working within health care induces different levels of stress in professionals. When dealing with life-limited children these stresses can be immense and, if not managed correctly, can lead to burnout.

# Issues

The issues that health care professionals may face involve the following.[1]

- Their own feelings around advancing disease and death, and the impact this work has on the practitioners and their family.
- Their ability to recognize, reflect on, and deal with conflicts of belief and values within the team.
- Their ability to work to resolve conflicts when they arise.
- Their ability to recognize and manage their own personality, reactions, and emotions constructively in relation to self, patients, and colleagues.
- Their ability to manage anger.
- Their ability to give and receive criticism constructively.
- Their ability to manage uncertainty, the unexpected, make difficult decisions, and multitask.
- Their ability to recognize stress, mental ill health, and burnout in self and other professionals.
- Their ability to ask for help and hand over to others appropriately and their ability to use a range of methods to receive support from, and give support to, colleagues.
- Their ability to recognize and deal competently with potential sources of difficulty including:
  - over-involvement;
  - personal identification;
  - negative feelings and personality clashes;
  - demands that cannot be met.
- Effective time management and the ability to prioritize effectively.

# Management

The key to successful management of these issues is awareness of the problems and pre-planning of the solutions.

- It is important to have communication and support mechanisms built into any organization.
- The health care professional should know their capabilities through the process of reflective practice and discussion with colleagues.
- There should be an openness to consult other professionals to seek advice.
- Realistic goals and expectations need to be set when planning care for a child.
- The doctor, team, and family need to understand that, by definition of a terminal illness, treatments may fail and need to be adjusted continually.
- Parental reactions to the death of a child are very varied. Occasionally the parents need to vent these emotions and this is sometimes directed towards a health care professional. This should not be seen as a personal attack, but more of a reflection of the frustration the parent is feeling at the time. It can be helpful to ask the question 'how can we help these parents' rather than labelling them as being awkward.
- Team working can be difficult and team dynamics change over time. It is helpful to understand the theory of team building to understand that conflict can be a positive influence in building a team.
- Organizational culture should develop where criticism is seen as a positive opportunity to address issues and raise standards and not negatively to put people down. This can only happen if feedback is given in a constructive, respectful, and honest way.
- The professional should consider having a mentoring system to allow for an opportunity to discuss issues. If a formal system is not available then having an equal colleague who one can talk to informally can be helpful.
- All organizations should have a system of debrief after the death of a child. This allows the team to share an outlet of emotions in a controlled environment. This debrief needs to be led by an experienced member of the team.
- It is important to have built into the structure of any team an independent occupational health facility and also anonymous direct access to counselling.
- To be emotionally affected by the death of a child and even cry a few tears is normal; conversely, just because someone does not cry does not mean they have not been moved by the experience. However, to lose emotional control completely is damaging to the individual, their colleagues, and the family. Sadly, once we finish with one child there is always a list of others waiting for our professional input.
- Paediatric palliative care cannot be done in a hurry. The average palliative care assessment takes 1–2 hours. For the parents, the fact that their child is dying makes them a priority over everything and everyone else when things are going wrong. Any attempt to hurry

the consultation or to 'fob them off' is perceived very badly and is a
particularly common complaint.

- Once a health care professional reaches a stage of feeling overloaded
  the system should allow them to step back from front line work to
  recharge.
- Paediatric palliative care is not easy and is not something every
  professional can do. When it becomes apparent that an individual
  cannot face the emotional impact of this type of work, they should be
  allowed to leave without any sense of failure.

## Reference

**1** Educational Subgroup of the British Society of Paediatric Palliative Medicine and the Association of Children's Hospice Doctors (2008). *Curriculum in paediatric palliative medicine*, pp. 82–4. BSPPM and Association of Children's Hospice Doctors. Available for download from  www.act.org.uk.

# Education and training

# Background

By definition, a curriculum comprises:
- a set of competencies in the subject;
- a set of tools to evaluate them.

## Competencies

Formal and systematic training is essential if gaps in knowledge, skills, and attitude are to be recognized and rectified by those working, or hoping to work, in children's palliative care. Thorough training in medical care of sick children (e.g. completion of core paediatric Specialist Registrar training) is a prerequisite[1] but is not sufficient in itself.

### Adult palliative medicine curriculum

This forms the core of all specialist palliative medicine training, even in children. Some competencies are:
- common to adult and paediatric specialties (e.g. WHO Pain Ladder);
- modifiable to become relevant to paediatrics (e.g. opioid pharmacology);
- largely irrelevant to the paediatric specialty (e.g. management of breast cancer);
- omitted from the adult curriculum, but essential to the paediatric one.

Important omissions are:
- management of sick children;
- management of symptoms in some specific conditions (e.g. hypoxic ischaemic encephalopathy, cerebral palsy);
- developmental issues (psychological, emotional, physical);
- other omissions of which even those working in children's palliative care themselves may not be aware.[2]

### Modifications to the adult curriculum[3]
- Much can be imported into the paediatric subspecialty, forming the nucleus of a paediatric curriculum.
- Some material can be modified to become relevant to children, e.g. establishing a starting dose for morphine based on weight rather than age.
- Removal of irrelevant material.
- Introduction of relevant material from other paediatric subspecialty curriculums (e.g. community paediatrics, neurodisability).
- Introduction of material signposted by the *Compendium of paediatric palliative care*.[4]
- Introduction of competencies suggested by research among children's hospice doctors.[2]

### Curriculum in paediatric palliative medicine

A curriculum for paediatric palliative medicine was developed in this way by the Education and training subgroup of the British Society for Paediatric Palliative Medicine.[5] This has formed the basis for:
- a formal curriculum in the subspecialty of PPM, approved by the Postgraduate Medical Education and Training Board (PMETB);
- a more detailed informal teaching guide for trainers in recognized PPM training posts;

- an informal curriculum for GPs working in children's hospices (in consultation with the Association for Children's Hospice Doctors.

The generic curriculum is available for download from ✍ www.act.org.uk.

## Evaluation tools

Evaluation tools for training in paediatric subspecialties is dictated by PMETB approval of the entire paediatric curriculum. This is available from ✍ www.rcpch.ac.uk.

Evaluation tools specific to the subspecialty of palliative medicine include:

- communication skills assessment by observation and video;
- structured portfolio of case reports;
- relevant clinical audits;
- structured examination questions.

## Levels of training

In paediatric palliative medicine, four levels of competence are currently described.

- Level 1 (expected from all newly qualified doctors). Understand basic principles of palliative care.
- Level 2 (expected of all those completing their core paediatric training). Apply basic principles to the care of children, and recognize reversible causes.
- Level 3 (consultant paediatrician with special interest in palliative medicine). Be able to manage most common symptoms, but recognize need to consult tertiary specialist when appropriate.
- Level 4 (tertiary specialist in paediatric palliative medicine). Have completed 2 year national grid training programme in paediatric palliative medicine.

It is anticipated that there will be parallel levels for general practitioners working in children's hospices. The extent to which the two curriculums can or should diverge is currently being considered by a joint working group of the BSPPM and the Association for Children's Hospice Doctors.

**Summary**

- Paediatric palliative medicine was recognized as a subspecialty of paediatrics in 2009
- The intention of developing a curriculum is not simply to recognize what is already done, but to set a standard for improvement
- Unusually among paediatric subspecialties, PPM is defined by the need of patients, rather than by their diagnosis or diseased organ system (which may indeed not be known)
- Children's hospices require palliative care skills for children rooted both in primary care and in paediatrics. This interface with primary care is an important and unique part of PPM training

## References

1 Hain, R. and Goldman, A. (2003). Training in paediatric palliative medicine. *Palliat. Med.* **17** (3), 229–31.

2 Amery, J. and Lapwood, S. (2004). A study into the educational needs of children's hospice doctors: a descriptive quantitative and qualitative survey. *Palliat. Med.* **18** (8), 727–33.

3 Hain, R, Rawlinson, F., and Finlay, I. (2004). 'A paediatric option?' The diploma in palliative medicine 3 years on. *Arch. Dis. Child.* **89** (S1), A35.

4 Children's International Project on Palliative/Hospice Services (2001). *Compendium of pediatric palliative care programs and practices.* National Hospice and Palliative Care Organization, Alexandria, Virginia.

5 Hain, R., Jassal, S., Rajapakse, D., McCulloch, R., and Lapwood, S. (2008). *Curriculum in paediatric palliative medicine.* British Society of Paediatric Palliative Medicine, Cardiff.

# Formulary

# Introduction

This formulary includes doses used in palliative care as those recommended in the BNFC. Readers outside the UK are advised to consult local prescribing guidelines (where they exist) as well.

# Amitriptyline

**Use** Neuropathic pain.

### Dose and routes

By mouth:
- child 2–12 years, initially 200–500mcg/kg (max. 25mg) once daily at night increased if necessary: max. 1mg/kg twice daily on specialist advice;
- child 12–18 years, initially 10–25mg once daily at night, increased gradually if necessary to 75mg at night.

### Notes

- Unlicensed for use with children with neuropathic pain.
- Comes in tablets (10mg, 25mg, 50mg) and oral solution (25mg/5mL, 50mg/5mL).

# Arthrotec®

**Use** Anti-inflammatory pain killer. For musculoskeletal pain and bone pain caused by tumour. Prophylaxis against NSAID-induced gastroduodenal ulceration in patients requiring diclofenac.

### Dose and routes[1]

By mouth:
- Arthrotec® 50, 1 tablet 2–3 times a day.
- Arthrotec® 75, 1 tablet 2 times a day.

### Notes

- Unlicensed for children.
- Above doses only for adults.
- Comes in tablets.

# Aspirin

**Use** Mild to moderate pain. Pyrexia.

### Dose and routes

By mouth:
- > 16 years of age, 300–900 mg every 4–6h when necessary: max. 4g daily.

### Notes
- Comes in tablets (75mg, 300mg), dispersible tablets (75mg, 300mg), and suppositories (150mg).

# Baclofen

**Use** Chronic severe spasticity of voluntary muscle.

### Dose and routes
By mouth:
- initially: child 1–10 years, 0.75–2mg/kg daily or 2.5mg 4 times daily;
- increased gradually to maintenance:
  - child 1–2 years, 10–20mg daily in divided doses;
  - child 2–6 years, 20–30mg daily in divided doses;
  - child 6–10 years, 30–60mg in divided doses.

### Notes
- Unlicensed for children < 1 year old.
- Avoid abrupt withdrawal.
- Comes in tablets (10mg) and oral solution (5mg/5mL).

# Bisacodyl

**Use** Constipation.

### Dose and routes
By mouth:
- child 4–10 years, 5mg at night;
- child 10–18 years, 5–10mg at night: increased if necessary (20mg).

By rectum (suppository):
- child 2–10 years, 5mg in the morning;
- child 10–18 years, 10mg in the morning.

### Notes
- Tablets act in 10–12h. Suppositories act in 20–60min.
- Comes in tablets (5mg) and suppositories (5mg, 10mg).

# Buprenorphine

**Use** Moderate to severe pain.

### Dose and routes

By sublingual route:
- child body weight 16–25kg, 100mcg every 6–8 hours;
- child body weight 25–37.5kg, 100–200mcg every 6–8 hours;
- child body weight 37.5–50kg, 200–300mcg every 6–8 hours;
- child body weight over 50kg, 200–400mcg every 6–8 hours.

By transdermal patch:

By titration or as indicated by existing opioid needs.

### Notes
- Sublingual tablets not licensed for use in children < 6 years old.
  - Comes in tablets (200mcg, 400mcg).
- Patches unlicensed in children. Two types of patches:
  - BuTrans®—applied every 7 days. Comes as 5 (5mcg/h for 7 days), 10 (10mcg/h for 7 days), and 20 (20mcg/h for 7 days);
  - TransTec®—applied every 96 hours. Comes as 35 (35mcg/hh for 96h), 52.5 (52.5mcg/hh for 96h), and 70 (70mcg/h for 96h).

# Carbamazepine

**Use** Neuropathic pain. Some movement disorders.

### Dose and routes

By mouth:
- child 1 month–12 years
  - initially 5mg/kg at night or 2.5mg/kg twice daily, increased as necessary by 2.5–5mg every 3–7 days;
  - usual maintenance dose 5mg/kg 2–3 times daily; doses up to 20mg/kg have been used.
- child 12–18 years
  - initially 100–200mg 1–2 times daily;
  - increased slowly to usual maintenance of 400–600mg 2–3 times daily.

By rectum:
- Child 1 month–18 years, use approximately 25% more than the oral dose (max. 250mg) up to 4 times a day.

### Notes
- Unlicensed for use with children with neuropathic pain.
- Can cause serious blood, hepatic, and skin disorders. Parents should be taught how to recognize signs of these conditions, particularly leucopenia.
- Different preparations may vary in bioavailability so avoid changing formulations.
- Comes in tablets (100mg, 200mg, 400mg), chewtabs (100mg, 200mg), liquid (100mg/5mL), suppositories (125mg, 250mg), and modified release tablets (200mg, 400mg).

# Chloral hydrate

**Use** Insomnia.

## Dose and routes

By mouth or rectum:
- child 0–12 years, 30–50mg/kg single dose at night;
- child 12–18 years, 0.5–1g single dose at night.

## Notes

- Oral use: mix with plenty of juice, water, or milk to reduce gastric irritation and disguise the unpleasant taste.
- For rectal administration use oral solution or suppositories made on manufacturer's special license.
- Accumulates on prolonged use and should be avoided in severe renal or hepatic impairment.
- Comes in tablets (cloral betaine 707mg = cloral hydrate 414mg—Welldorm®), oral solution (143.3mg/5mL—Welldorm®, 200mg/5mL, 500mg/5mL).

# Clonazepam

**Use** Tonic-clonic seizures, partial seizures, myoclonus, and status epilepticus.

## Dose and routes

By mouth:
- child 1 month–1 year, initially 250mcg at night for 4 nights, increased over 2–4 weeks to usual maintenance dose of 0.5–1mg at night (may be given in 3 divided doses if necessary);
- child 1–5 years, initially 250mcg at night for 4 nights, increased over 2–4 weeks to usual maintenance of 1–3mg at night (may be given in 3 divided doses if necessary);
- child 5–12 years, initially 500mcg at night for 4 nights, increased over 2–4 weeks to usual maintenance dose of 3–6mg at night (may be given in 3 divided doses if necessary);
- child 12–18 years, initially 1mg at night for 4 nights, increased over 2–4 weeks to usual maintenance of 4–8mg at night (may be given in 3 divided doses if necessary).

## Notes

- Comes in tablets (500mcg, 2mg) and oral solution (2.5mg/mL, other strengths as 'specials').
- Tablets licensed in children. Oral liquid unlicensed in UK.

# Co-danthramer

**Use** Constipation in terminal illness only.

### Dose and routes

By mouth:
- co-danthramer 25/200 suspension 5mL = one co-danthramer 25/200 capsule:
  - child 2–12 years, 2.5–5mL at night;
  - child 6–12 years, 1 capsule at night;
  - child 12–18 years, 5–10mL or 1–2 capsules at nightl
- strong co-danthramer 75/1000 suspension 5mL = two strong co-danthramer 37.5/500 capsules:
  - child 12–18 years, 5mL or 1–2 capsules at night.

### Notes

- Co-danthramer is made from danthron and poloxamer '188'.
- Avoid prolonged skin contact due to risk of irritation and excoriation.
- Rodent studies indicate potential carcinogenic risk.

# Co-danthrusate

**Use** Constipation in terminal illness only.

### Dose and routes

By mouth:
- child 6–12 years, 5mL or 1 capsule at night;
- child 12–18 years, 5–15mL or 1–3 capsules at night.

### Notes

- Co-danthrusate is made from danthron and docusate sodium.
- Avoid prolonged skin contact due to risk of irritation and excoriation.
- Rodent studies indicate potential carcinogenic risk.

# Codeine phosphate

**Use** Mild to moderate pain.

### Dose and routes

By mouth, rectum, sc injection, or by im injection:
- neonate, 0.5–1mg/kg every 4–6h;
- child 1 month–12 years, 0.5–1mg/kg every 4–6h, max. 240mg daily;
- child 12–18 years, 30–60mg every 4–6h, max. 240mg daily.

### Notes

- Unlicensed for use with children < 1 year old.
- Rectal administration is an unlicensed route.
- ▶ Must *not* be given iv.
- Reduce dose in renal impairment.
- Comes in tablets (15mg, 30mg, 60mg), oral solution (25mg/5mL), and injection (60mg/mL).

# Cyclizine

**Use** Nausea and vomiting if cause is intracerebral.

## Dose and routes

By mouth or by slow iv injection over 3–5min:

- child 1 month–6 years, 0.5–1mg/kg up to 3 times daily, max. single dose 25mg;
- child 6–12 years, 25mg up to 3 times daily;
- child 12–18 years, 50mg up to 3 times daily.

By rectum:
child 2–6 years, 12.5mg up to 3 times daily;
child 6–12 years, 25mg up to 3 times daily;
child 12–18 years, 50mg up to 3 times daily.

By continuous iv or sc infusion:
child 1 month-6 years, 3mg/kg over 24h;
child 2–5 years, 50mg over 24h;
child 6–12 years, 75mg over 24h;
child 12–18 years, 150mg over 24h,

## Notes

- Tablets may be crushed for oral administration.
- Tablets not licensed for use in children < 6 years old.
- Injection not licensed for use in children.
- Comes in tablet (50mg), suppositories (12.5mg, 25mg, 50mg, 100mg by 'special' order), and injection (50mg/mL).

# Dantrolene

**Use** Skeletal muscle relaxant. Chronic severe muscle spasm or spasticity.

**Dose and routes**

By mouth:
- child 5–12 years, initially 500mcg/kg once daily; after 7 days increase to 500mcg/kg/dose 3 times daily. Every 7 days increase by further 500mcg/kg/dose until response. Max. 2mg/kg 3–4 times daily (max. total daily dose 400mg).
- child 12–18 years, initially 25mg once daily; after 7 days increase to 25mg 3 times daily. Every 7 days increase by further 500mcg/kg/dose until response. Max. 2mg/kg 3–4 times daily (max. total daily dose 400mg).

**Notes**
- Unlicensed for use with children for this indication.
- Comes in capsules (25mg, 100mg), oral solution (can be extemporaneously prepared).

# Dexamethasone

**Use**
- Headache associated with raised intracranial pressure caused by tumour.
- Anti-inflammatory in brain and other tumours causing pressure on nerves or bone.
- Antiemetic either as an adjuvant or in highly emetogenic cytotoxic therapies.

**Dose and routes**

*Headache associated with raised intracranial pressure*

By mouth or iv: child 1 month–12 years, 250mcg/kg twice a day for 5 days; then reduce or stop if possible.

*To relieve symptoms of brain or other tumour*

Numerous other indications in palliative medicine, only in discussion with specialist palliative medicine team.

*Antiemetic*

By mouth or iv:
- child < 1 year, 250mcg–1mg 3 times daily;
- child 1–5 years, 1–2mg 3 times daily;
- child 6–12 years, 2–4mg 3 times daily;
- child 12–18 years, 4mg 3 times daily.

**Notes**
- Unlicensed for use with children as antiemetic.
- Dexamethasone 1mg = dexamethasone phosphate 1.2mg = dexamethasone sodium phosphate 1.3mg.
- Tablets may be dispersed in water or injection solution given by mouth.

- Comes in tablets (500mcg, 2mg), oral solution (as specials 500mcg/5mL, 2mg/5mL), and injection (4mg/1mL).
- Weight gain and other serious side effects with long-term use.

# Diazepam

### Use
- Short term anxiety relief.
- Relief of muscle spasm.
- Treatment of status epilepticus.

### Dose and routes

#### Short term anxiety relief[2]
By mouth:
- child 2–12 years, 2–3mg 3 times daily;
- child 12–18 years, 2–10mg 3 times daily.

#### Relief of muscle spasm
By mouth:
- child 1–12 months, initially 250mcg/kg twice a day;
- child 1–5 years, initially 2.5mg twice a day;
- child 5–12 years, initially 5mg twice a day;
- child 12–18 years, initially 10mg twice a day, max. Total daily dose 40mg.

#### Status epilepticus
By iv injection over 3–5min:
- neonate, 300–400mcg/kg repeated after 10min if necessary;
- child 1 month–12 years, 300–400mcg/kg repeated after 10min if necessary;
- child 12–18 years, 10–20mg repeated after 10min if necessary.

By rectum (rectal solution):
- neonate, 1.25–2.5mg repeated after 10min if necessary;
- child 1 month–2 years, 5mg repeated after 10min if necessary;
- child 2–12 years, 5–10mg repeated after 10min if necessary;
- child 12–18 years, 10mg repeated after 10min if necessary.

### Notes
- Comes in tablets (2mg, 5mg, 10mg), oral solution (2mg/5mL, 5mg/5mL), rectal tubes (2.5mg, 5mg, 10mg, 20mg), and injection (5mg/mL).
- Rectal tubes not licensed for children < 1 year old.

# Diclofenac

**Use** Mild to moderate pain and inflammation, particularly musculoskeletal disorders.

## Dose and routes

By mouth or rectum:
- child 6 months–18 years, 0.3–1mg/kg (max. 50mg) 3 times daily.

By im or iv injection:[2]
- child 6 months–18 years, 0.3–1mg/kg 1–2 times a day max. of 150mg/day and for a max. 2 days.

## Notes
- Unlicensed for use with children < 1 year old.
- Suppositories unlicensed for use with children < 6 years old (except in children > 1 year old with juvenile idiopathic arthritis).
- Injections unlicensed for use with children.
- Diclofenac potassium unlicensed for use with children < 14 years old.
- Solid forms of 50mg or more unlicensed for use with children.
- Comes in tablets/capsules (25mg, 50mg, 75mg modified release), dispersible tablets (10mg, 50mg), and injection (25mg/mL).

# Docusate

**Use** Constipation.

## Dose and routes

By mouth:
- child 6 months–2 years, initially 12.5mg 3 times daily;
- child 2–12 years, initially 12.5–25mg 3 times daily;
- child 12–18 years, up to 500mg daily in divided doses.

By rectum:
- child 12–18 years, 1 enema as single dose.

## Notes
- Adult oral solution and capsules not licensed in children < 12 years.
- Oral preparations act within 1–2 days.
- Rectal preparations act within 20min.
- Doses may be exceeded on specialist advice.
- Comes in capsules (100mg), oral solution (12.5mg/5mL paediatric, 50mg/5mL adult), and enema (120mg in 10g single dose pack).

# Domperidone

## Use
- Nausea and vomiting where poor GI motility is the cause.
- Gastro-oesophageal reflux resistant to other therapy.

## Dose and routes

By mouth:
- body-weight ≤ 35kg, initially 250–500mcg/kg 3–4 times daily, max. 2.4mg/kg in 24h;
- body-weight > 35kg, initially 10–20mg 3–4 times daily, max. 80mg/24h.

By rectum:
- body-weight 15–35kg, 30mg twice a day;
- body-weight > 35kg, 60mg twice a day.

## Notes

- Only licensed in children for the management of nausea and vomiting following radiotherapy or chemotherapy.
- Comes in tablets (10mg), oral solution (5mg/5mL), and suppositories (30mg).

# Entonox (nitrous oxide)

**Use** As self-regulated analgesia without loss of consciousness. Particularly useful for painful dressing changes.

## Dose and routes

By inhalation:
- child usually > 5 years old, self-administration using a demand valve. Up to 50% in oxygen according to child's needs.

## Notes

- Is normally used as a light anaesthesia.
- Should only be used as self-administration using a demand valve; all other situations require specialist paediatric anaesthetist.
- Is dangerous in the presence of pneumothorax or intracranial air after head injury.
- Prolonged use can cause megaloblastic anaemia.

# Erythromycin

**Use** Gastrointestinal stasis (motilin receptor agonist).

## Dose and routes

By mouth:
- neonate, 3mg/kg 4 times daily;
- child 1 month–18 years, 3mg/kg 4 times daily.

## Notes

- Unlicensed for use with children with gastrointestinal stasis.
- Comes in tablets (250mg, 500mg) and oral solution (125mg/5mL, 250mg/5mL).

# Etamsylate

**Use** Treatment of haemorrhage.

**Dose and routes**[1]
By mouth:
- > 18 years, 500mg 4 times daily.

**Notes**
- Unlicensed for use with children with haemorrhage.
- Comes in tablets (500mg).

# Fentanyl

**Use** Step 3 WHO pain ladder once dose is titrated.

**Dose and routes**
By transmucosal application (lozenge with oromucosal applicator):
- Child 2–18 years, 15–20mcg/kg as a single dose, max. dose 400mcg.

By transdermal patch:
- based on oral morphine dose equivalent (given at 24-hour totals).
  Product monograph:
  - oral morphine 60–134mg = 25mcg/h patch of fentanyl;
  - oral morphine 180–224mg = 50mcg/h patch of fentanyl;
  - oral morphine 270–314mg = 75mcg/h patch of fentanyl.

**Notes**
- Unlicensed for use with children.
- If using more than 4 doses of lozenges for breakthrough pain then adjust background analgesia.
- Comes in lozenge (200mcg, 400mcg, 600mcg, 800 mcg, 1.2mg, 1.6mg) and patches ('12', '25', '50', '75', '100'mcg/h).

# Fluoxetine

**Use** Major depression.

**Dose and routes**
By mouth:
- child 12–18 years, 10mg once a day, max. 20mg once daily.

**Notes**
- Unlicensed for use with children.
- Use with caution in children ideally with specialist advice.
- Comes in capsules (20mg) and oral solution (20mg/5mL).

# Gabapentin

**Use** Adjuvant in neuropathic pain.

### Dose and routes

By mouth:
- Child 2–6 years, initially 10mg/kg increasing gradually according to response to usual dose 30–60mg/kg in 3 divided doses.
- Child 6–12 years, initially 10mg/kg (max. 300mg) increasing gradually according to response to usual dose 25–35mg/kg in 3 divided doses.
- Child 12–18 years, initially 300mg increasing gradually according to response to usual dose 0.9–3.6g in 3 divided doses.

### Notes

- Unlicensed for use with children with neuropathic pain.
- No consensus on dose for neuropathic pain. Doses given based on doses for partial seizures and authors' experience.
- Capsules can be opened but have a bitter taste.
- Comes in capsules (100mg, 300mg, 400mg), tablets (600mg, 800mg).

# Gaviscon®

**Use** Gastro-oesophageal reflux, dyspepsia, and heartburn.

### Dose and routes

By mouth:
- neonate–2 years, body weight < 4.5kg, 1 dose (half dual sachet) when required, max. 6 times in 24h;
- neonate–2years body weight > 4.5kg, 2 doses (1 dual sachet) when required, max. 6 times in 24h;
- child 2–12 years, 2.5–5mL or 1 tablet after meals and at bedtime;
- child 12–18 years, 5–10mL or 1–2 tablet after meals and at bedtime.

**Notes** Comes in tablets, liquid (Gaviscon® Advance), and infant sachets (comes as dual sachets, each half of dual sachet is considered one dose).

# Glycerol (glycerin)

**Use** Constipation.

### Dose and routes

By rectum:
- child 1 month–1 year, 1g suppository as required;
- child 1–12 years, 2g suppository as required;
- child 12–18 years, 4g suppository as required.

### Notes

- Moisten with water before insertion.
- Comes in suppository (1g, 2g, 4g).

# Glycopyrronium bromide

**Use** Control of upper airways secretion and hypersalivation.

**Dose and routes** By mouth: child 1 month-18 years, 40–100mcg/kg 3–4 times daily.

**Notes**

- Unlicensed for use with children for control of upper airways secretion and hypersalivation.
- For oral administration injection solution may be given or crushed tablets suspended in water.
- Comes in tablets (1mg, 2mg on named patient basis) and injection (200mcg/mL).

# Haloperidol

**Use**

- Nausea and vomiting where cause is metabolic.
- Restlessness and confusion.
- Intractable hiccups.

**Dose and routes**

By mouth for nausea and vomiting:
- child 12–18 years, 1.5mg once daily at night, increased to 1.5mg twice a day, max. 5mg twice a day.

By mouth for restlessness and confusion:
- child dose dependent on weight, 10–20mcg/kg every 8–12h.

By mouth for intractable hiccups:
- child 12–18 years, 1.5mg 3 times daily.

By continuous iv or sc infusion (for any indication):
- child 1 month–12 years, 25–85mcg/kg over 24h;
- child 12–18 years, 1.5–5mg over 24h.

**Notes**

- Unlicensed for use with children with nausea and vomiting, or restlessness and confusion, or intractable hiccups.
- Comes in tablets (500mcg, 1.5mg, 5mg, 10mg, 20mg), capsules (500mcg), oral solution (1mg/mL, 2mg/mL), and injection (5mg/mL).

# Hydromorphone

**Use** Alternative opioid analgesic for severe pain (Step 3 WHO Pain Ladder).

**Dose and routes**

By mouth:
- child 12–18 years, initially 1.3mg every 4h increasing as required.

## Notes

- Licensed for use with children with cancer pain.
- Modified release capsules given 12 hourly.
- Capsules (both types) can be opened and contents sprinkled on soft food.
- Comes in capsules (1.3mg, 2.6mg) and modified release capsules (2mg, 4mg, 8mg, 16mg, 24mg).

# Hyoscine butylbromide

**Use** Adjuvant where pain is caused by spasm of the gastrointestinal or genitourinary tract.

## Dose and routes

By mouth:
- child 1 month–2 years, 300–500mcg/kg (max. 5mg) 3–4 times daily;
- child 2–5 years, 5mg 3–4 times daily;
- child 5–12 years, 10mg 3–4 times daily;
- child 12–18 years, 10–20mg 3–4 times daily.

By im or iv injection:
- child 1 month–4 years, 300–500mcg/kg (max. 5mg) 3–4 times daily;
- child 5–12 years, 5–10mg 3–4 times daily;
- child 12–18 years, 10–20mg 3–4 times daily.

## Notes

- Tablets unlicensed for use with children < 6 years old.
- Injection unlicensed for use with children.
- For administration by mouth, injection solution may be given. Injection solution can be stored for 24h in the refrigerator.
- iv injection should be given slowly over 1min and can be diluted with glucose 5% or sodium chloride 0.9%.
- Comes in tablets (10mg) and injection (20mg/mL).

# Hyoscine hydrobromide

**Use** Control of upper airways secretion and hypersalivation.

## Dose and routes

By mouth or sublingual:
- child 2–12 years, 10mcg/kg, max. 300mcg 4 times daily;
- child 12–18 years, 300mcg 4 times daily.

By transdermal route:
- child 1 month–3 years, quarter of a patch every 72h;
- child 3–10 years, half of a patch every 72h;
- child 10–18 years, one patch every 72h.

By sc or iv injection or infusion:
- child by weight, 10mcg/kg (max. 600mcg) every 4–8h.

## Notes
- Unlicensed for use with children for control of upper airways secretion and hypersalivation.
- Apply patch to hairless area of skin behind ear.
- Patches are often cut for titration.
- For administration by mouth injection solution may be given.
- Comes in tablets (150mcg), patches (1mg/72h), and injection (400mcg/mL, 600mcg/mL).

# Ibuprofen

**Use** Simple analgesic and adjuvant for musculoskeletal pain.

## Dose and routes

By mouth:
- child 1–3 months, 5mg/kg 3–4 times daily preferably after food;
- child 3–6 months, 50mg 3 times daily preferably after food; in severe conditions up to 30mg/kg daily in 3–4 divided doses;
- child 6 months–1 year, 50 mg 3–4 times daily preferably after food; in severe conditions up to 30 mg/kg daily in 3–4 divided doses;
- child 1-4 years, 100 mg 3 times daily preferably after food; in severe conditions up to 30 mg/kg daily in 3–4 divided doses;
- child 4–7 years, 150 mg 3 times daily, preferably after food. In severe conditions, up to 30mg/kg daily in 3–4 divided doses. Maximum daily dose, 2.4g;
- child 7–10 years, 200mg 3 times daily, preferably after food. In severe conditions, up to 30mg/kg daily in 3–4 divided doses. Max. daily dose, 2.4g;
- child 10–12 years, 300mg 3 times daily, preferably after food. In severe conditions, up to 30mg/kg daily in 3–4 divided doses. Maximum daily dose, 2.4g;
- > 12 years—see adult dose.

Pain and inflammation in rheumatic diseases, including idiopathic juvenile arthritis:
- children aged 3 months–8 years and body weight > 5kg, 30–40mg/kg daily in 3–4 divided doses preferably after food up to a maximum of 2.4g daily;
- in systemic juvenile idiopathic arthritis, up to 60mg/kg daily in 4–6 divided doses up to a maximum of 2.4g daily (unlicensed).

### Notes
- Topical preparations and granules unlicensed for use with children.
- Liquid and plain tablets unlicensed for use with children < 7kg or < 1 year old.
- Comes in tablets (200mg, 400mg, 600mg), capsule (300mg MR), oral solution (100mg/5mL), spray, creams, gels (5%), and granules (600mg/sachet).

# Ketamine

**Use** Adjuvant for neuropathic pain.

### Dose and routes
By mouth or sc infusion: 0.1–0.3 mg/kg/h (max. 1.5mg/kg/h).

### Notes
- Unlicensed for use with children with neuropathic pain.
- Specialist use only.
- Comes in injection (10mg/mL, 50mg/mL, 100mg/mL) and oral solution special preparation.

# Levomepromazine

### Use
- Antiemetic where cause is unclear, or where probably multifactorial.
- Second line if specific antiemetic fails.

### Dose and routes

*Used as antiemetic*

By mouth:
- child 2–12 years, starting dose 0.1–1mg/kg, max 25mg;
- child > 12 years, 6.25–25mg by mouth once or twice daily.

By continuous iv or sc infusion over 24h:
- child 1 month–12 years, 100–400mcg/kg over 24h;
- child 12–18 years, 5–25mg over 24h.

*Used for sedation*

By sc infusion over 24h:
- child 1 year–12 years, 0.35–3mg/kg over 24h;
- child 12–18 years, 12.5–200mg over 24h.

*Analgesia*
- May be of benefit in a very distressed patient with severe pain unresponsive to other measures.
- Stat dose 0.5mg/kg by mouth or sc. Titrate dose according to response; usual maximum daily dose in adult 100mg sc or 200mg by mouth.

### Notes
- Unlicensed for use with children for these indications.
- For sc infusion dilute with sodium chloride 0.9%.
- Can cause hypotension particularly with higher doses.
- Comes in tablets (25mg) and injection (25mg/mL).

# Lidocaine

### Use Neuropathic pain.

### Dose and routes
By patch: 5% patches available. Maximum recommended number of patches in adults currently is 3.

### Notes
- Unlicensed for use with children with neuropathic pain.
- Comes in patch (5%).

# Lomotil® (co-phenotrope)

### Use Diarrhoea from non-infectious cause.

### Dose and routes

By mouth:
- child 2–4 years, half tablet 3 times daily;
- child 4–9 years, 1 tablet 3 times daily;
- child 9–12 years, 1 tablet 4 times daily;
- child 12–16 years, 2 tablets 3 times daily;
- child 16–18 years, initially 4 tablets then 2 tablets 4 times daily.

### Notes

- Unlicensed for use with children < 4 years.
- Co-phenotrope (2.5mg diphenoxylate hydrochloride and 25mcg atropine sulphate).
- Tablets may be crushed.
- Comes in tablet only.

# Loperamide

**Use** Diarrhoea from non-infectious cause.

### Dose and routes

By mouth:
- child 1 month–1 year, 100–200mcg/kg twice daily, 30min before feeds; up to 2mg/kg daily in divided doses;
- child 1–12 years, 100–200mcg/kg (max. 2mg) 3–4 times daily; up to 1.25mg/kg daily in divided doses (max. 16mg daily);
- child 12–18 years, 2–4mg 2–4 times daily (max. 16mg daily).

### Notes

- Unlicensed for use with children with chronic diarrhoea.
- Capsules unlicensed for use with children < 8 years.
- Syrup unlicensed for use with children < 4 years
- Comes in capsules/tablets (2mg) and oral solution (1mg/5mL).

# Lorazepam

## Use
- Background anxiety.
- Adjuvant in cerebral irritation.
- Background management of dyspnoea.
- Muscle spasm.

## Dose and routes
By mouth:
- child < 2 years, 25mcg/kg 2–3 times daily;
- child 2–5 years, 0.5mg 2–3 times daily;
- child 6–10 years, 0.75mg 3 times daily;
- child 11–14 years, 1mg 3 times daily;
- child 15–18 years, 1–2mg 3 times daily.

## Notes
- Unlicensed for use with children for these indications.
- Comes in tablet (1mg).

# Melatonin

**Use** Sleep disturbance due to disruption of circadian rhythm (▶ *not anxiolytic*).

## Dose and routes
By mouth:
- dose unknown, but the following has been used: initially 2–3mg, increasing every 1–2 weeks dependent on effectiveness up to max. 10mg (higher doses have been used).

## Notes
- Unlicensed for use with children.
- Specialist use only.
- Comes in various formulations dependent on source.

# Methadone

**Use** Major opioid (step 3), particularly in neuropathic pain.

## Dose and routes
Dose unknown, but following doses have been used.

### Used as breakthrough with other major opioid as background
By mouth:
- child 2–12 years, 0.1–0.2mg/kg as needed 4 hourly;
- child 12–18 years, 3–5mg as needed 4 hourly.

*Used in opioid substitution*
- There is no single agreed approach or opioid equivalency. Local specialist palliative medicine guidelines should be cited.
- Dangers of sudden overdose (secondary peak phenomenon) so rotation to methadone should only be undertaken on inpatients.
- Caution: rotation to methadone is a specialist palliative medicine skill and should only be undertaken in close collaboration with the local specialist team. There is a risk of unexpected death through overdose.

### Notes
- Unlicensed for use with children with neuropathic pain.
- Use of methadone complicated by variable equivalency with other opioids, and by idiosyncratic distribution that can result in sudden toxicity (secondary peak phenomenon).
- Use only under specialist palliative medicine or pain advice.
- Close supervision and monitoring are required when commencing regular use.
- Current practice in adults is usually to admit to a specialist inpatient unit for first 1–2 weeks of regular treatment.
- Comes in linctus (2mg/5mL), mixture (1mg/mL), solution (1mg/mL, 10mg/mL, 20mg/mL), tablets (5mg), and injection (10mg/mL).

# Metoclopramide

### Use
- Antiemetic if vomiting caused by gastric compression or hepatic disease.
- Prokinetic for slow transit time (not in complete obstruction or with anticholinergics)

### Dose and routes
By mouth, im injection, or iv injection:
- neonate, 100 mcg/kg every 6–8h (by mouth or iv only);
- child 1 month–1 year and body weight up to 10kg, 100mcg/kg (max. 1mg) twice daily.
- child 1–3 years and body weight up to 10–14kg, 1mg 2–3 times daily;
- child 3–5 years and body weight up to 15–19kg, 2mg 2–3 times daily;
- child 5–9 years and body weight up to 20–29kg, 2.5mg 3 times daily;
- child 9–10 years and body weight up to 30–60kg, 5mg 3 times daily;
- child 15–18 years and body weight over 60kg, 10mg 3 times daily.

### Notes
- Unlicensed for use with neonates as prokinetic.
- Comes in tablets (10mg), oral solution (5mg/5mL), and injection (5mg/mL).

# Metronidazole topically

**Use** Odour associated with fungating wound or lesion.

### Dose and routes
By topical application:
- apply to clean wound 1–2 times daily and cover with non-adherent dressing;
- cavities: smear gel on paraffin gauze and pack loosely.

### Notes
- Anabact® not licensed for use in children < 12 years.
- Metrogel® not licensed for use with children.
- Comes in gel (Anabact® 0.75%, Metrogel® 0.75%, Metrotop 0.8%).

# Micralax® Micro-enema (sodium citrate)

**Use** Constipation where osmotic laxative indicated.

### Dose and routes
By rectum: child 3–18 years, 5mL as a single dose.

### Notes
- Not recommended in children < 3 years.
- Comes in micro-enema (5mL).

# Midazolam

### Use
- Status epilepticus and terminal seizure control.
- Breakthrough' anxiety, e.g. panic attacks.
- Adjuvant for pain of cerebral irritation.
- Dyspnoea.

### Dose and routes
By buccal administration for status epilepticus:
- neonate, 300mcg/kg as a single dose;
- child 1–6 months, 300mcg/kg (max. 2.5mg), repeated once if necessary;
- child 6 months–1 year, 2.5mg, repeated once if necessary;
- child 1–5 years, 5mg, repeated once if necessary;
- child 5–10 years, 7.5mg, repeated once if necessary;
- child 10–18 years, 10mg, repeated once if necessary.

By sc or iv infusion over 24h for anxiety or terminal seizure control: 50–300mcg/kg/h. Doses above 80mg in 24h are usually unnecessary and can lead to paradoxical agitation.

### Notes
- Unlicensed for use with children with these conditions.
- Comes in oral solution (2.5mg/mL), buccal liquid (10mg/mL), and injection (1mg/mL, 2mg/mL, 5mg/mL).

# Morphine

**Use** Major opioid (step 3). First line oral opioid for breakthrough and background.

### Dose and routes
By mouth:
- child 1–12 months, initially 80–200mcg/kg every 4h adjusted to response;
- child 1–2 years, initially 200–400mcg/kg every 4h adjusted to response;
- child 2–12 years, initially 200–500mcg/kg (max. 20mg) every 4h adjusted to response;
- child 12–18 years, initially 5–20mg every 4h adjusted to response.

By continuous sc infusion:
- child 1–3 months, 10mcg/kg/h adjusted to response;
- child 3 months–18 years, 20mcg/kg/h adjusted to response.

Parenteral dose 50% of oral dose.

### Notes
- Oramorph® solution not licensed for use with children < 1 year.
- Oramorph® unit dose vials not licensed for use with children < 6 years.
- Sevredol® tablets not licensed for use with children < 3 years.
- Where opioid substitution or rotation is to morphine: use oral morphine equivalency (OME; see Chapter 7, Introduction).
- Comes in:
  - tablets (10mg, 20mg, 50mg);
  - oral solution (10mg/5mL, 30mg/5mL, 100mg/5mL);
  - modified release tablets (5mg, 10mg, 15mg, 30mg, 60mg, 100mg, 200mg);
  - modified release suspension (20mg, 30mg, 60mg, 100mg, 200mg);
  - suppositories (10mg, 15mg, 20mg, 30mg);
  - injection (10mg, 15mg, 20 mg and 30mg).

# Movicol®

### Use
- Constipation.
- Faecal impaction.
- Suitable for opioid-induced constipation.

### Dose and routes (Movicol® paediatric plain)
By mouth for constipation:
- child 1–6 years, 1 sachet daily (max. 4 sachets daily);
- child 6–12 years, 2 sachets daily (max. 4 sachets daily);
- child 12–18 years, 1–3 sachets daily of adult Movicol®.

By mouth for faecal impaction:
- child 1–5 years, 2 sachets on first day and increase by 2 sachets every 2 days (max. 8 sachets daily);
- child 5–12 years, 4 sachets on first day and increase by 2 sachets every 2 day (max. 12 sachets daily);
- child 12–18 years, 8 sachets daily of adult Movicol® for max. 3 days.

### Notes
- Unlicensed for use with children < 5 years with faecal impaction and < 2 years with chronic constipation.
- Mix powder with water: Movicol® paediatric 60mL/sachet and adult Movicol® 125mL/sachet.

# Nabilone

### Use
Antiemetic if vomiting caused by anxiety/anticipation (e.g. chemotherapy).

### Dose and routes
By mouth: adult dose, 1–2mg twice a day as required.

### Notes
- Unlicensed for use with children.
- Comes in capsules (1mg).

# Naloxone

### Use
Constipation when caused by opioids.

### Dose and routes
By mouth. In adults the following doses have been used: total daily dose oral naloxone = 20% of morphine dose; titrate according to need; max. single dose 5mg.

### Notes
- Unlicensed for use with children with constipation.
- Although oral availability of naloxone is relatively low, be alert for opioid withdrawal symptoms, including recurrence of pain, at higher doses.
- Comes in injection (400mcg/mL).

# Omeprazole

### Use
- Gastro-oesophageal reflux.
- Treatment of peptic ulcers.
- Gastrointestinal prophylaxis (e.g. with combination NSAID/steroids).

### Dose and routes
By mouth:
- neonate, 700mcg/kg once daily, max. 2.8mg/kg daily;
- child 1 month–2 years, 700mcg/kg once daily, max. 3mg/kg daily;
- child body weight 10–20kg, 10mg once daily max. 20mg for 12 weeks;
- child body weight > 20kg, 20mg once daily max. 40mg for 12 weeks.

### Notes
- Unlicensed for use with children except for severe ulcerating reflux oesophagitis in children > 1 year.
- For oral administration tablets can be dispersed in water or 10mL sodium bicarbonate 8.4%. Capsules can be opened and mixed with fruit juice or yoghurt.
- Comes in tablets (10mg, 20mg, 40mg) and capsules (10mg, 20mg, 40mg).

# Ondansetron

### Use
- Antiemetic, if vomiting caused by chemotherapy or radiotherapy.
- Vomiting breaking through background levomepromazine

### Dose and routes
By mouth:
- Child 1–12 years, 4mg by mouth every 8–12h for up to 5 days after chemotherapy.
- Child 12–18 years, 8mg by mouth every 8–12h for up to 5 days after chemotherapy.

### Notes
- Unlicensed for use with children < 2 years.
- Comes in tablets (4mg, 8mg), oral lyophilisates (4mg, 8mg), and oral solution (4mg/5mL).

# Oxygen

### Use
- Dyspnoea caused by hypoxaemia.
- Placebo in other causes of dyspnoea.

# Pamidronate

### Use
- Bone pain caused by metastatic disease or osteopenia.
- Acute hypercalcaemia.

### Dose and routes
- For bone pain (metastatic bone disease or osteopenia): 1mg/kg infused over 6h, repeated daily for 3 days. Can be given 3 monthly.
- For malignant hypercalcaemia: 1mg/kg infused over 6h, then repeated as indicated by serum calcium.

### Notes
- Unlicensed for use with children.
- Many bisphosphonates available in different formulations, including oral. Risk of osteonecrosis, especially of jaw if pre-existing pathology.
- Anecdotal risk of iatrogenic osteopetrosis with prolonged use (if prolonged use likely, precede with DEXA scan and investigation of calcium metabolism).

# Phenobarbital

### Use
- Adjuvant in pain of cerebral irritation.
- Control of terminal seizures.
- Sedation.

### Dose and routes
By mouth:
- neonates, loading dose by slow iv injection, then 20mg/kg by mouth once a day;
- child 1 month–12 years, 1–1.5mg/kg twice a day, increased by 2mg/kg daily as required (usual maintenance dose 2.5–4mg/kg once or twice a day;
- child 12–18 years, 60–180mg once a day.

### Notes
- Tablets may be crushed.
- Comes in tablets (15mg, 30mg, 60mg) and oral solution (15mg/5mL).

# Quinine

**Use** Leg cramps.

## Dose and routes

By mouth:
- not licensed or recommended for children as no experience;
- adult dose 200–300mg at night.

## Notes
- Unlicensed for use with children for this condition.
- Comes in tablets (200mg, 300mg).

# Ranitidine

## Use
- Gastro-oesophageal reflux.
- Treatment of peptic ulcers.
- GI prophylaxis (e.g. with combination NSAID/steroids)

## Dose and routes

By mouth:
- neonate, 2–3mg/kg body weight of ranitidine 3 times daily;
- child 1–6 months, 1mg/kg body weight 3 times daily to max. 3mg/kg body weight 3 times daily;
- child 6 months–3 years, 2–4mg/kg body weight twice a day;
- child 3–12 years, 2–5mg/kg body weight (max. single dose 300mg) twice a day;
- child 12–18 years, 150mg twice a day or 300mg at night. May be increased if necessary in moderate to severe gastro-oesophageal reflux disease to 300mg twice a day or 150mg 4 times daily, for up to 12 weeks.

## Notes
- Unlicensed for use with children < 3 years.
- Comes in tablets (150mg, 300mg) and oral solution (75mg/5mL).

# Temazepam

**Use** Sleep disturbance where anxiety is a cause.

## Dose and routes

By mouth: adult, 10–40mg at night.

## Notes
- Unlicensed for use with children.
- Comes in tablets (10mg, 20mg) and oral solution (10mg/5mL).

# Tizanidine

**Use** Muscle spasm.

**Dose and routes**

Adult dose:
- initially 2mg increasing in increments of 2mg at intervals of 3–4 days;
- give total daily dose in divided doses up to 3–4 times daily;
- usual total daily dose 24mg; Max. total daily dose 36mg.

**Notes**
- Unlicensed for use with children.
- Timing of dose individual to specific patient as maximal effect is seen after 2–3h and is short-lived.
- Usually prescribed and titrated by neurologists.
- Comes in tablets (2mg, 4mg).

# Tramadol

**Use** Minor opioid (step 2) with additional non-opioid analgesic actions.

**Dose and routes**

By mouth: child 12–18 years, initially 50mg every 4–6h, max. 400mg/day.

**Notes**
- Unlicensed for use with children < 12 years.
- Although a minor opioid, additional non-opioid effects mean OME more than might be expected.
- May be appropriate to consider small doses of morphine for breakthrough when background is tramadol.
- Comes in tablets (50mg, 100mg), capsules (50mg, 100mg), and soluble tablets (50mg).

# Tranexamic acid

**Use** Oozing of blood (e.g. from mucous membranes), particularly when due to low or dysfunctional platelets.

**Dose and routes**

By mouth: child 1 month–12 years, 15–25mg/kg (max. 1.5g) 2–3 times daily.

**Notes**
- Parenteral preparation can be used topically.
- Comes in tablets (500mg).

# Triclofos

**Use** Sleep disturbance. Not anxiolytic or analgesic.

### Dose and routes
By mouth:
- neonate, 25–30mg/kg at night;
- child 1 month–1 year, 25–30mg/kg at night;
- child 1–5 years, 250–500mg at night;
- child 6–12 years, 0.5–1g at night;
- child 12–18 years, 1–2g at night.

### Notes
- Unlicensed for use with children with neuropathic pain.
- Comes as oral solution (500mg/5mL).

# Ventolin® (salbutamol)

**Use** Dyspnoea where reversible bronchospasm is a cause.

### Dose and routes
By nebulized solution: child 1 month–18 years, 2.5–5mg up to 4 times daily.

**Notes** Comes in nebulizer solution (2.5mg, 5mg).

## References

**1** British Medical Association (2008). *British national formulary* (BNF). BMJ Publishing Group, RPS Publishing, London.

**2** Royal College of Paediatrics and Child Health (2003). *Medicines for children*, 2nd edn. RCPCH Publications Ltd, London.

**3** Jassal, S. (2007). *Basic symptom control in paediatric palliative care, the Rainbows Children's Hospice guidelines*, 7th edn. Rainbows Children's Hospice, Loughborough.

# Index

Entries in **bold** indicate formulary information.